QUALITATIVE RESEARCH
IN HEALTH CARE
Second edition

QUALITATIVE RESEARCH IN HEALTH CARE

Second edition

Edited by

CATHERINE POPE
*Lecturer in Medical Sociology, Department of Social
Medicine, University of Bristol, England*

and

NICHOLAS MAYS
*Health Adviser, Social Policy Branch,
The Treasury, Wellington, New Zealand*

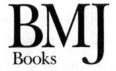

BMJ
Books

© BMJ Books 2000
BMJ Books is an imprint of the BMJ Publishing Group
www.bmjbooks.com

First published in 1996
by the BMJ Publishing Group, BMA House, Tavistock Square,
London WC1H 9JR

First edition 1996
Second impression 1997
Second edition 1999
Second impression 2001

British Library Cataloguing in Publication Data

A catalogue record for this book is available from the British Library

ISBN 0-7279-1396-4

Typeset by Apek Typesetters, Nailsea, Bristol
Printed and bound in Great Britain by JW Arrowsmith Ltd, Bristol

Contents

List of contributors   vii

Preface   ix

1 Qualitative methods in health research   1
CATHERINE POPE, NICHOLAS MAYS

2 Qualitative interviews in health care research   11
NICKY BRITTEN

3 Focus groups with users and providers of health care   20
JENNY KITZINGER

4 Observational methods in health care settings   30
CATHERINE POPE, NICHOLAS MAYS

5 Using the Delphi and nominal group technique in
health services research   40
JEREMY JONES, DUNCAN HUNTER

6 Using case studies in health services and
policy research   50
JUSTIN KEEN, TIM PACKWOOD

7 Using qualitative methods in health-related
action research   59
JULIENNE MEYER

8 Analysing qualitative data   75
CATHERINE POPE, SUE ZIEBLAND, NICHOLAS MAYS

9 **Quality in qualitative health research** 89
NICHOLAS MAYS AND CATHERINE POPE

Index 103

List of contributors

Nicky Britten, *senior lecturer in medical sociology, GKT Department of General Practice, King's College, London*

Duncan Hunter, *assistant professor, Community Health and Epidemiology, Queen's University, Kingston, Ontario, Canada*

Jeremy Jones, *lecturer in health economics, Nuffield Community Care Studies Unit, Department of Epidemiology and Public Health, University of Leicester, Leicester*

Justin Keen, *fellow in health systems, King's Fund, London*

Jenny Kitzinger, *reader in sociology, Department of Human Sciences, Brunel University, Middlesex*

Nicholas Mays, *health adviser, Social Policy Branch, The Treasury, Wellington, New Zealand*

Julienne Meyer, *professor of adult nursing, City University, London*

Tim Packwood, *senior lecturer in public and social administration, Department of Government, Brunel University, Middlesex*

Catherine Pope, *lecturer in medical sociology, Department of Social Medicine, University of Bristol, Bristol*

Sue Ziebland, *senior research fellow, ICRF GP Research Group, Institute of Health Sciences, University of Oxford, Oxford*

Preface to the second edition

We were unaware, when we presented our Socratic dialogue about qualitative methods to the 1991 Society for Social Medicine Annual Scientific Meeting, just what we were getting ourselves into. Our tongue-in-cheek fictional argument between a qualitative sociologist and the medical director of a health services research unit was conceived as a comment on the apparent failure of those studying health and health care to understand the potential contribution of qualitative methods (which had such a long, fruitful history in anthropology, medical sociology and educational research). These methods – based on interviews and observation – were largely unfamiliar to many health professionals and researchers. Indeed, they seemed alien alongside the traditionally accepted methods of experimental science and statistical analysis.

A version of our dialogue was published subsequently in the *British Medical Journal*[1] and led first to a commissioned series of papers in the Journal and then, in 1996, to the first edition of this book. Since writing that first paper, there has been a big expansion in qualitative health services research in the UK and a growing enthusiasm for an "exciting range of qualitative methods capable of providing basic understanding of the process and outcomes of health care".[2] Editorials in leading medical journals have extolled the virtues of qualitative methods, and reports of studies using these methods have appeared in those same journals.[3-6] In revising this book we were reminded just how far qualitative research in health care has come, in a comparatively short space of time.

In compiling the enlarged second edition, our brief was to update the chapters with recent examples of research and new developments in the field of qualitative research on health. We have also taken the opportunity afforded by a more generous word limit to discuss some of the important theoretical and methodological issues that could not be tackled in the original papers and book. We have also attempted to incorporate and respond to constructive advice from colleagues, criticisms of reviewers, and pleas for more examples of qualitative research from health and research practitioners and teachers.

We wish to thank the colleagues and friends who have encouraged us and engaged us in methodological debate (and, crucially, told us when we have got it wrong). In this, special thanks are due to Professor Nick Black and Dr David Hughes, who carefully peer-reviewed the first edition for us and made useful suggestions for this new volume. Chapter 9 draws heavily on the invaluable systematic review of applied qualitative methods by Murphy and colleagues,[7] and their timely publication of this review was much appreciated. As ever, we owe a huge debt of thanks to the authors of the chapters and we are grateful for the assistance of the editorial team at BMJ Books, not least Mary Banks, who rose to the challenge of dealing with editors on opposite sides of the globe.

Catherine Pope and Nicholas Mays
1999

1 Pope C, Mays N. Opening the black box: an encounter in the corridors of health services research. *Br Med J* 1993;**306**:315–8.
2 Fitzpatrick R, Boulton M. Qualitative methods for assessing health care. *Quality in Health Care* 1994;**3**:107–13 (quote at 112).
3 Anon. Population health looking upstream. *The Lancet* 1994;**343**:429–30.
4 Black N. Why we need qualitative research. *Journal of Epidemiology and Community Health* 1994;**48**:425–6.
5 Scheff T, Starrin B. Qualitative methods in the health sciences. *European Journal of Public Health* 1997;**7**:355–6.
6 Popay J, Rogers A, Williams G. Qualitative research and the gingerbread man. *Health Education Journal* 1995;**54**:389–92.
7 Murphy E, Dingwall R, Greatbach D, Parker S, Watson P. Qualitative research methods in health technology assessment: a review of the literature. *Health Technology Assessment* 1998:**2**(16).

1 Qualitative methods in health research

CATHERINE POPE, NICHOLAS MAYS

Qualitative research methods have long been used in the social sciences. They are the principal methods employed by anthropologists to study the customs and behaviours of peoples from other cultures, and they are also used in such diverse areas as sociology, semiotics, psychology, education, history and cultural studies. Qualitative methods have much to offer those studying health and health care settings, and they are increasingly being used in health services research. However, because these methods have traditionally been employed in the social sciences, they may be unfamiliar to health care professionals and researchers with biomedical or natural science backgrounds. Indeed, qualitative methods may seem alien alongside the experimental and quantitative methods used in clinical, biological and epidemiological research. Misunderstandings about the nature of qualitative methods and their uses have meant that qualitative research is often labelled "unscientific". A frequent criticism is that qualitative data are necessarily subjective (and, therefore, biased) and that such research is difficult to replicate and amounts to little more than anecdote, personal impression or conjecture. This book seeks to counter this view. It aims to introduce some of the main qualitative methods and to indicate how they may be employed appropriately and fruitfully to answer some of the increasingly complex questions confronting health and health care researchers.

The link between theory and method

Misunderstandings about qualitative research may be compounded by some of the terminology used, which again, may be

1

unfamiliar to researchers with non-social science backgrounds. The terms "qualitative research" and "qualitative methods" are often used interchangeably, but, strictly speaking, *research methods* refer to specific research techniques used to gather data about the social world (such as questionnaires in survey research, or focus groups, discussed in Chapter 3). The choice of research method is typically informed by a *research strategy* or a set of decisions about the research design and by beliefs about how the social world can be studied and how the validity of social knowledge established by such research might be assessed. For many social scientists the choice of a particular research method is also inextricably linked to a particular *theoretical perspective* or set of explanatory concepts that provide a framework for thinking about the social world and inform their research (see Box 1).

Box 1—Some theoretical perspectives that inform qualitative methods[1,2]

- Ethnography
- Symbolic interactionism
- Constructionism
- Ethnomethodology
- Phenomenology

As a result of these different theoretical positions, qualitative research is neither unified nor well defined. There is considerable debate about what constitutes the central tenets of qualitative research. So, for example, Silverman[3] reviews four "definitions" of qualitative research before writing his own prescriptive account of what qualitative research should be. Elsewhere, Hammersley[4] has examined the methodological ideas which underlie the distinctive Chicagoan tradition of qualitative research, with its emphasis on *naturalistic methods* (see page 4). The debate about qualitative research is such that Denzin and Lincoln in their *Handbook of Qualitative Research*[5] are forced to conclude that it is "defined primarily by a series of essential tensions, contradictions and hesitations". The distinctions between the various theoretical stances are frequently presented as clear cut, but in practice the contrasts are often less apparent. Moreover, the connection between research and theoretical perspective may not always be clear: sometimes the link is implicit or simply not acknowledged.

So, while many social scientists contend that research should be theoretically driven, others have suggested that the link between theory and methods is overstated. Brannen, for example, has argued that "the practice of research is a messy untidy business which rarely conforms to the models set down in methodology textbooks. In practice it is unusual, for example, for epistemology or theory to be the sole determinant of method... There is no necessary or one-to-one correspondence between epistemology and methods".[6] She suggests that the choice of method and how it is used is as likely to be informed by the research question or pragmatic or technical considerations as by the researcher's theoretical stance (though others would disagree). This may be particularly the case in health services research because of its applied nature: research here tends to be geared towards specific practical problems or issues and this, rather than theoretical leanings, may determine the methods employed.

So what is qualitative research?

Qualitative research is often defined by reference to quantitative research. Its methods are seen as the antithesis of quantitative or statistical ones; indeed, the articles in the *British Medical Journal* on which the first edition of this book was based were commissioned, not as a series about qualitative research, but as a series on "non-quantitative methods". An unfortunate corollary of this way of defining qualitative research is the inference that because qualitative research does not seek to quantify or enumerate, it does not "measure". It is worth noting that it is both feasible and legitimate to analyse certain types of qualitative data quantitatively (see Chapter 8). Whilst it is true that qualitative research generally deals with talk or words rather than numbers, this does not mean that it is devoid of measurement, or that it cannot be used to explain social phenomena.

Measurement in qualitative research is usually concerned with *taxonomy* or classification. Qualitative research answers questions such as, "what is X, and how does X vary in different circumstances, and why?" rather than "how big is X or how many Xs are there?" It is concerned with the meanings people attach to their experiences of the social world and how people make sense of that world. It therefore tries to interpret social phenomena (interactions, behaviours, etc.) in terms of the meanings people bring to

3

them; because of this it is often referred to as *interpretative* research. This approach means that the researcher frequently has to question common sense assumptions or taken for granted ideas. Bauman,[7] talking about sociology in general, refers to this as "defamiliarising" and this is just what qualitative research tries to do. Rather than simply accepting the concepts and explanations used in everyday life, qualitative research asks fundamental and searching questions about the nature of social phenomena. So, for example, instead of counting the number of suicides, which presumes that we already agree on the nature of suicide, the researcher asks, "what is suicide?" and shows that it is socially constructed by the activities of coroners, legal experts, health professionals and individuals so that definitions of suicide vary considerably between different countries, different cultures and religious groups, and across time.[8]

A second distinguishing feature of qualitative research, and one of its key strengths, is that it studies people in their natural settings rather than in artificial or experimental ones. Kirk and Miller define qualitative research as a "particular tradition in social science that fundamentally depends on watching people in their own territory, and interacting with them in their own language, on their own terms".[9] This is referred to as *naturalism* – hence the term *naturalistic methods* sometimes used to denote the approach used in much, but not all, qualitative research.

Another feature of qualitative research (which some authors emphasise) is that it often employs several different methods or adopts a "multi-method" approach. Watching people in their own territory thus entails observing, joining in (*participant observation*), talking with people (interviews, focus groups and informal chatting) and reading what they have written. In the health care context, a range of qualitative research methods has been employed to tackle important questions about social phenomena, ranging from complex human behaviours such as patients' compliance with treatment,[10] and decision making by health care professionals,[11] through to the organisation of the hospital clinic[12] or of the NHS itself.[13,14]

Qualitative research, thus defined, appears very different from quantitative research. Much is made of the differences between the two. The so called qualitative–quantitative divide is often reinforced by highlighting a corresponding split in the social sciences between social theories concerned with delineating social structure and those concerned with understanding social action or meaning.[15, 16] The crude alignment of qualitative research with "action" or interpretive approaches and quantitative research with "structural" or positivist ones has meant that researchers on either side have tended to become locked into adversarial positions, ignorant of each other's work. The differences between qualitative and quantitative research are, as a result, frequently overstated, and this has helped to perpetuate the misunderstanding of qualitative methods within such fields as health services research.[17] However, there is a growing recognition within sociology that the qualitative–quantitative distinction may not be helpful or even accurate.[18,19] This perception appears to be gradually filtering through to health and health services research where qualitative and quantitative methods are increasingly being used together to answer research questions.[20]

The uses of qualitative research

Instead of seeing quantitative and qualitative approaches as methodological opposites, each can be used to complement the other. One simple way in which this can be achieved is by using qualitative research as the preliminary to quantitative research. This model is likely to be the most familiar to those engaged in health and health services research. For example, qualitative research can classify phenomena, or answer the "what is X?" question, which necessarily precedes the process of enumeration of Xs. As health care deals with people and people are, on the whole, more complex than the subjects of the natural sciences, there is a whole set of such questions about human interaction, and how people interpret interaction, to which health professionals may need answers before attempting to quantify behaviours or events. At their most basic, qualitative research techniques can be used simply to discover the most comprehensible terms or words in common use to include in a subsequent survey questionnaire. An excellent example of this can be found in the preliminary work undertaken for the British national survey of sexual attitudes and lifestyles.[21] In this case, face-to-face interviews were used to uncover popular ambiguities and misunderstandings of a number of terms such as "vaginal sex", "oral sex", "penetrative sex" and "heterosexual". This qualitative work had enormous value in informing the development of the subsequent survey questionnaire, and in ensuring the validity of the data obtained because

5

the language in the questionnaire was clear and could be widely understood.

Qualitative research is not only useful as the first stage of quantitative research. It also has a role to play in "validating" quantitative research or in providing a different perspective on the same social phenomena. Sometimes it can force a major reinterpretation of quantitative data. For example, one anthropological study using qualitative methods uncovered the severe limitations of previous surveys: Stone and Campbell found that cultural traditions and unfamiliarity with questionnaires led Nepalese villagers to feign ignorance of abortion and family planning services and to under-report their use of contraception and abortion when responding to surveys.[22] More often, the insights provided by qualitative research help us to interpret or understand quantitative data more fully. Bloor's work on the surgical decision making process built on an epidemiological study of the widespread variations in rates of common surgical procedures (see Box 2) and helped to unpack the reasons why these variations occurred.[11] Elsewhere, Morgan and Watkin's research on cultural beliefs about hypertension has helped to explain why rates of compliance with prescribed medications vary significantly amongst and between white and Afro-Caribbean patients.[10]

As well as complementing quantitative work, qualitative research may also be used quite independently to uncover social processes, or access areas of social life which are not open or amenable to quantitative research. This type of "stand alone" qualitative research is increasingly being used in studies of health service organisation and policy. It has been used to considerable effect in evaluating organisational reforms and changes to health service provision from the viewpoint of patients, health professionals and managers.[14, 23] This type of research has also been useful in examining how data about health and health care are shaped by the social processes that produce them – from waiting lists[24] to death certificates[25] and AIDS registrations.[26]

Methods used in qualitative research

Qualitative research explores people's subjective understandings of their everyday lives. Although the different disciplines use qualitative methods in slightly different ways, broadly speaking, the methods used in qualitative research include direct observation, interviews, the analysis of texts or documents and of recorded speech or behaviour (audio/video tapes). Data collected by these methods may be used differently (for example, semiotics and psychotherapy both use video and/or audio-taped material but their analytical approaches are distinctive), but there is a common focus on talk and action rather than numbers. On one level, these "qualitative methods" are used every day by human beings to make sense of the world – we watch what is going on, ask questions of each other and try to comprehend the social world we live in. The

---

Box 2—Two stage investigation of the association between differences in geographic incidence of operations on the tonsils and adenoids and local differences in specialists' clinical practices[27]

I Epidemiological study—documenting variations
Analysis of 12 months' routine data on referral, acceptance, and operation rates for new patients under 15 years in two Scottish regions known to have significantly different 10 year operation rates for tonsils and adenoids.

Found significant differences between similar areas within regions in referral, acceptance, and operation rates that were not explained by disease incidence.

Operation rates influenced, in order of importance, by:

• Differences between specialists in propensity to list for operations
• Differences between GPs in propensity to refer
• Differences between areas in symptomatic mix of referrals

II Sociological study—explaining how and why variations come about
Observation of assessment routines undertaken in outpatient departments by six consultants in each region on a total of 493 under 15s.

Found considerable variation between specialists in their assessment practices (search procedures and decision rules), which led to differences in disposals, which in turn created local variations in surgical incidence.

"High operators" tended to view a broad spectrum of clinical signs as important and tended to assert the importance of examination findings over the child's history; "low operators" gave the examination less weight in deciding on disposal and tended to judge a narrower range of clinical features as indicating the need to operate.

key difference between this and the qualitative methods employed in social science is that the latter are systematic. Qualitative research, therefore, involves the application of logical, planned and thorough methods of collecting data, and careful, thoughtful and, above all, rigorous analysis. As several recent commentators have pointed out, this means that qualitative research requires considerable skill on the part of the researcher.[28,29] Perhaps more than some quantitative research techniques, qualitative research needs experienced researchers. One of the problems arising from the rapid expansion of qualitative methods into medical and health fields is that the necessary skill and experience are sometimes lacking.

This book focuses on three main methods: face-to-face interviews, focus groups (or group discussions) and observation. We have chosen to concentrate on these three methods because they appear to be the most widely used in health and health services settings. Thus, the scope of the book is necessarily restricted. We have neglected some methods, for example, documentary methods and textual analysis,[30] which have been used, for example, to describe media reporting of AIDS[31] and the public and professional attitudes to tranquilliser use engendered by the popular press.[32] We have also not looked at conversation analysis in health research.[33] The book is introductory and aims to show how these three methods can be appropriately and fruitfully employed in health research. It seeks to provide clear examples of these methods and to indicate some of the benefits and common pitfalls in their use. It is not a substitute for seeking the advice of a skilled, experienced researcher, nor is it an exhaustive manual for qualitative research. In addition to the references, which provide a route to more detailed material on each of the topics covered, each chapter ends with a short guide to further reading.

Following the three chapters devoted to specific methods, we have included a section looking at how these methods have been applied in health research. Our aim here is simply to demonstrate how qualitative methods may be used. We have deliberately chosen three areas (consensus development, case studies and action research) where qualitative methods are currently being used in health and health services research. It is not our intention to argue that these approaches are synonymous with qualitative research, but rather to indicate how qualitative methods have fruitfully been employed in these ways. Chapter 8 deals with the analysis of the textual data generated by the three methods and, because of their widespread use, we have included a description of some of the software packages currently available to assist this process. The concluding chapter reviews the place of qualitative methods in health research and examines the issue of "quality" in qualitative research, and how it may be assessed.

Further reading

Gubruim J, Holstein J. *The new language of qualitative method.* New York: Oxford University Press, 1997.
Murphy E, Dingwall R, Greatbatch D, Parker S, Watson P. Qualitative research methods in health technology assessment: a review of the literature. *Health Technology Assessment* 1998;2(16) (see section 1).

References

1 Marshall C, Rossman G. *Designing qualitative research.* London: Sage, 1989.
2 Feldman MS. *Strategies for interpreting qualitative data.* Qualitative Research Methods Series, No 33. Thousand Oaks, CA: Sage, 1995.
3 Silverman D. *Interpreting qualitative data: methods for analysing talk, text and interaction.* London: Sage, 1993.
4 Hammersley M. *The dilemma of qualitative method: Herbert Blumer and the Chicago tradition.* London: Routledge, 1989.
5 Denzin NK, Lincoln YS, eds. *Handbook of qualitative research.* London: Sage, 1994:ix.
6 Brannen J, ed. *Mixing methods: qualitative and quantitative research.* Aldershot: Avebury, 1992:3, 15.
7 Bauman Z. *Thinking sociologically.* Oxford: Blackwell, 1990.
8 Douglas J. *The social meanings of suicide.* Princeton, NJ: Princeton University Press, 1967.
9 Kirk J, Miller M. *Reliability and validity in qualitative research.* Qualitative Research Methods Series, No 1. London: Sage, 1986:9.
10 Morgan M, Watkins C. Managing hypertension: beliefs and responses to medication among cultural groups. *Sociology of Health and Illness* 1988;10:561–78.
11 Bloor M. Bishop Berkeley and the adenotonsillectomy enigma: an exploration of the social construction of medical disposals. *Sociology* 1976;10:43–61.
12 Strong PM. *The ceremonial order of the clinic.* London: Routledge, 1979.
13 Strong PM, Robinson J. *The NHS: Under new management.* Milton Keynes: Open University Press, 1990.
14 Pollitt C, Harrison S, Hunter D, Marnoch G. General management in the NHS: the initial impact, 1983–88. *Public Administration* 1991;69:61–83.
15 Mechanic D. Medical sociology: some tensions among theory, method and substance. *Journal of Health and Social Behavior* 1989;30:147–60.
16 Pearlin L. Structure and meaning in medical sociology. *Journal of Health and Social Behavior* 1992;33:1–9.
17 Pope C, Mays N. Opening the black box: an encounter in the corridors of health services research. *Br Med J* 1990;306:315–18.
18 Abell P. Methodological achievements in sociology over the past few decades with special reference to the interplay of qualitative and quantitative methods.

In: Bryant C, Becker H, eds. *What has sociology achieved?* London: Macmillan, 1990.

19 Hammersley M. Deconstructing the qualitative–quantitative divide. In Brannen J, ed. *Mixing methods: qualitative and quantitative research.* Aldershot: Avebury, 1992.

20 Barbour R. The case for combining qualitative and quantitative approaches in health services research. *Journal of Health Services Research and Policy* 1999;4:39–43.

21 Wellings K, Field J, Johnson A, Wadsworth J. *Sexual behaviour in Britain: the national survey of sexual attitudes and lifestyles.* Harmondsworth: Penguin, 1994.

22 Stone L, Campbell JG. The use and misuse of surveys in international development: an experiment from Nepal. *Human Organisation* 1986;43:27–37.

23 Packwood T, Keen J, Buxton M. *Hospitals in transition: the resource management experiment.* Milton Keynes: Open University Press, 1991.

24 Pope C. Trouble in store: some thoughts on the management of waiting lists. *Sociology of Health and Illness* 1991;13:191–211.

25 Prior L, Bloor M. Why people die: social representations of death and its causes. *Science as culture* 1993;3:346–74.

26 Bloor M, Goldberg D, Emslie J. Ethnostatistics and the AIDS epidemic. *British Journal of Sociology* 1991;42:131–7.

27 Bloor MJ, Venters GA, Samphier ML. Geographical variation in the incidence of operations on the tonsils and adenoids: an epidemiological and sociological investigation. *J Laryngol Otol* 1976;92:791–801, 883–95.

28 Malterud K. Shared understanding of the qualitative research process: guidelines for the medical researcher. *Family Practice* 1993;10:201–6.

29 Dingwall R, Murphy E, Watson P, Greatbatch D, Parker S. Catching goldfish: quality in qualitative research. *Journal of Health Services Research and Policy* 1998;3:167–72.

30 Plummer K. *Documents of life: an introduction to problems and literature of a humanistic method.* London: Allen and Unwin, 1983.

31 Kitzinger J, Miller D. "African AIDS": the media an audience believes. In: Aggleton P, Davies P, Hart G, eds. *AIDS: Rights, risk and reason.* London: Falmer Press, 1992.

32 Gabe J, Gustaffson U, Bury M. Mediating illness: newspaper coverage of tranquilliser dependence. *Sociology of Health and Illness* 1991;13:332–53.

33 Goodwin C, Heritage J. Conversation analysis. *Annual Review of Anthropology* 1990;19:283–307.

2 Qualitative interviews in health care research

NICKY BRITTEN

Interviews are the most commonly used qualitative technique in health care settings. The attraction of interview-based studies for practising clinicians is their apparent proximity to the clinical task. However, this is also a danger as the many differences between clinical work and qualitative research may be overlooked.

Types of qualitative interview

Practising clinicians routinely interview patients during their clinical work, and they may wonder whether simply talking to people constitutes a legitimate form of research. In sociology and related disciplines, however, interviewing is a well-established research technique. There are three main types: structured, semistructured and depth interviews (see Box 1).

Structured interviews consist of administering structured questionnaires, and interviewers are trained to ask questions (mostly with a fixed choice of responses) in a standardised manner. For example, interviewees might be asked: "Is your health excellent,

---

Box 1—Types of interviews

- Structured
  Usually with a structured questionnaire
- Semistructured
  Open ended questions
- Depth
  One or two issues covered in great detail
  Questions are based on what the interviewee says

---

good, fair or poor?" Though qualitative interviews are often described as being unstructured in order to contrast them with this type of formalised interview designed to yield quantitative data, the term "unstructured" is misleading, as no interview is completely devoid of structure. If there were no structure, there would be no guarantee that the data gathered would be appropriate to the research question.

Semistructured interviews are conducted on the basis of a loose structure consisting of open-ended questions that define the area to be explored, at least initially, and from which the interviewer or interviewee may diverge in order to pursue an idea or response in more detail. Continuing with the same example, interviewees might initially be asked a series of questions such as: "What do you think good health is?", "How do you consider your own health?" and so on.

Depth interviews are less structured than this, and may cover only one or two issues, but in much greater detail. Such an interview might begin with the interviewer saying, "This research study is about how people think about their own health. Can you tell me about your own health experiences?" Further questions from the interviewer would be based on what the interviewee said, and would consist mostly of clarification and probing for details.

Interviews have been used extensively in studies of both patients and doctors. For example, Britten interviewed 30 attenders and non-attenders at two general practices to explore patients' ideas about medicines.[1] A semistructured interview schedule of 16 questions was used, but respondents were also encouraged to talk freely. The data revealed that on the one hand much medicine taking was taken for granted and, on the other hand, that patients had many fears and powerful negative images of medicines. Black and Thompson interviewed 28 consultants and 34 junior doctors about their perceptions of the role of medical audit.[2] Although the doctors accepted the need for audit, the study identified 19 obstacles to audit. In general, criticisms were levelled at the way audit was being implemented rather than at the underlying principles.

Clinical and qualitative research interviews have very different purposes. Although the doctor may be willing to see the problem from the patient's perspective, the clinical task is to fit that problem into an appropriate medical category in order to choose an appropriate form of management. The constraints of most consultations are such that any open-ended questioning needs to be brought to a conclusion by the doctor within a fairly short time. In a qualitative research interview, the aim is to discover the interviewee's own framework of meanings and the research task is to avoid imposing the researcher's structures and assumptions on the interviewee's account as far as possible. The research needs to remain open to the possibility that the concepts and variables that emerge may be very different from those that might have been predicted at the outset.

Qualitative interview studies address different questions from those addressed by quantitative research. For example, a quantitative epidemiological approach to the sudden infant death syndrome might measure statistical correlates of national and regional variations in incidence. In a qualitative study, by contrast, Gantley *et al.* interviewed mothers of young babies in different ethnic groups to understand their child rearing practices and hence discover possible factors contributing to the low incidence of sudden infant death in Asian populations.[3] A quantitative study of single-handed general practitioners might compare their prescribing and referral rates, out-of-hours payments, list sizes, and immunisation and cervical cytology rates with those of general practitioners in partnerships. A recent qualitative study used semistructured interviews to examine the concerns of single-handed general practitioners.[4] This research identified a range of problems perceived by this group of doctors, such as inadequate premises, difficulties finding locums and therefore with taking holidays, and difficulties with the general practitioner contract. Qualitative research can also open up different areas of research such as hospital consultants' views of their patients, or general practitioners' accounts of uncomfortable prescribing decisions.[5,6]

Conducting interviews

Qualitative interviewers try to be interactive and sensitive to the language and concepts used by the interviewee, and they try to keep the agenda flexible. They aim to go below the surface of the topic being discussed, explore what people say in as much detail as possible, and uncover new areas or ideas that were not anticipated at the outset of the research. It is vital that interviewers check that they have understood respondents' meanings instead of relying on their own assumptions. This is particularly important if there is

13

obvious potential for misunderstanding – for example, when a clinician interviews someone unfamiliar with medical terminology. Clinicians should not assume that interviewees use medical terminology in the same way that they do.

Patton has written that good questions in qualitative interviews should be open-ended, neutral, sensitive and clear to the interviewee.[7] He listed six types of questions that can be asked: those based on behaviour or experience, on opinion or value, on feeling, on knowledge, on sensory experience, and those asking about demographic or background details (see Box 2). It is usually best to start with questions that the interviewee can answer easily and then proceed to more difficult or sensitive topics. Most interviewees are willing to provide the kind of information the researcher wants, but they need to be given clear guidance about the amount of detail required. This way, it is possible to collect data even in stressful circumstances.[8]

Box 2—Types of questions for qualitative interview[7]

- Behaviour or experience
- Opinion or belief
- Feelings
- Knowledge
- Sensory
- Background or demographic

The less structured the interview, the less the questions are determined and standardised before the interview occurs. Most qualitative interviewers will have a list of core questions that define the areas to be covered, based on the objectives of their study. Unlike quantitative interviews based on highly structured questionnaires, the order in which questions are asked will vary, as will the questions designed to probe the interviewee's meanings. Wordings cannot be standardised because the interviewer will try to use the person's own vocabulary when framing supplementary questions. Also, during the course of a qualitative study, the interviewer may introduce further questions as he or she becomes more familiar with the topic being discussed.

All qualitative researchers need to consider how they are perceived by interviewees and the effects of personal characteristics such as class, race, sex and social distance on the interview. This question becomes more acute if the interviewee knows that the interviewer is also a doctor or nurse. An interviewee who is already a patient or likely to become one may wish to please the doctor or nurse by giving the responses he or she thinks the doctor or nurse wants. It is best not to interview one's own patients for research purposes, but if this cannot be avoided, patients should be given permission to say what they really think, and they should not be corrected if they say things that clinicians think are wrong (for example, that antibiotics are a suitable treatment for viral infections).

Interviewers are also likely to be asked questions by interviewees during the course of an interview. The problem with this is that in answering questions, clinical researchers may undo earlier efforts not to impose their own concepts on the interview. On the other hand, if questions are not answered, this may reduce the interviewee's willingness to answer the interviewer's subsequent questions. One solution is to say that such questions can be answered at the end of the interview, although this is not always a satisfactory response.[9]

Researcher as research instrument

Qualitative interviews require considerable skill on the part of the interviewer. Experienced doctors and other clinicians may feel that they already possess the necessary skills, and indeed many are transferable. To achieve the transition from consultation to research interview, clinical researchers need to monitor their own interviewing technique, critically appraising tape recordings of their interviews and asking others for their comments. The novice research interviewer needs to notice how directive he or she is being, whether leading questions are being asked, whether cues are picked up or ignored, and whether interviewees are given enough time to explain what they mean. Whyte devised a six point directiveness scale to help novice researchers analyse their own interviewing technique (see Box 3).[10] The point is not that non-directiveness is always best, but that the amount of directiveness should be appropriate to the style of research. Some informants are more verbose than others, and it is vital that interviewers maintain

---

Box 3—Whyte's directiveness scale for analysing interviewing technique[10]

1 Making encouraging noises
2 Reflecting on remarks made by the informant
3 Probing on the last remark by the informant
4 Probing an idea preceding the last remark by the informant
5 Probing an idea expressed earlier in the interview
6 Introducing a new topic
(1 = least directive, 6 = most directive)

---

control of the interview. Patton provided three strategies for maintaining control: knowing the purpose of the interview, asking the right questions to get the information needed, and giving appropriate verbal and non-verbal feedback (see Box 4).[7]

Holstein and Gubrium have written about the "active" interview to emphasise the point that all interviews are collaborative enterprises.[11] They argue that both interviewer and interviewee are engaged in the business of constructing meaning, whether this is acknowledged or not. They criticise the traditional view in which a passive respondent is accessing a "vessel of answers" that exists independently of the interview process. The interview is an active process in which the respondent activates different aspects of her or his stock of knowledge, with the interviewer's help. They conclude that an active interview study has two aims: "to gather information about *what* the research project is about and to explicate *how* knowledge concerning that topic is narratively constructed".

Some common pitfalls for interviewers identified by Field and Morse include outside interruptions, competing distractions, stage fright, awkward questions, jumping from one subject to another, and the temptation to counsel interviewees (see Box 5).[12] Awareness of these pitfalls can help the interviewer to develop ways of overcoming them, ranging from simple tasks such as unplugging

---

Box 4—Maintaining control of the interview[7]

• Knowing what it is you want to find out
• Asking the right questions to get the information you need
• Giving appropriate verbal and non-verbal feedback

Box 5—Common pitfalls in interviewing[12]

- Interruptions from outside (telephone, etc)
- Competing distractions (children, etc)
- Stage fright for interviewer or interviewee
- Asking interviewee embarrassing or awkward questions
- Jumping from one subject to another
- Teaching (for example, giving interviewee medical advice)
- Counselling (for example, summarising responses too early)
- Presenting one's own perspective, thus potentially biasing the interview
- Superficial interviews
- Receiving secret information (for example, suicide threats)
- Translators (for example, inaccuracy)

the telephone and rephrasing potentially embarrassing questions, through to conducting the interview at the interviewee's own pace and assuring the interviewee that there is no hurry.

Recording interviews

There are various ways of recording qualitative interviews: notes written at the time, notes written afterwards, and audio taping. Writing notes at the time can interfere with the process of interviewing, and notes written afterwards are likely to miss out some details. In certain situations, written notes are preferable to audio taping, but most people will agree to having an interview tape recorded, although it may take them a little while to speak freely in front of a machine. It is vitally important to use good quality equipment that has been tested beforehand and with which the interviewer is familiar. A good quality portable microphone can enhance the recording quality of a cheap tape recorder. Transcription is an immensely time consuming process, as each hour's worth of a one-to-one interview can take six or seven hours to transcribe, depending on the quality of the tape (and, as Chapter 3 explains, this transcription time increases considerably for group interviews). The costing of any interview-based study should include adequate transcription time.

Identifying interviewees

Sampling strategies should always be determined by the purpose of the research project.[12] Statistical representativeness is not normally sought in qualitative research.[13] Similarly, sample sizes are not determined by hard and fast rules, but by other factors, such as the depth and duration required for each interview and how much it is feasible for a single interviewer to undertake. Large qualitative studies do not often interview more than 50 or 60 people, although there are exceptions.[14] Sociologists conducting research in medical settings often have to negotiate access with great care, although this is unlikely to be a problem for clinicians conducting research in their own place of work. Nevertheless, the researcher still needs to approach the potential interviewee and explain the purpose of the research, emphasising that a refusal will not affect future treatment. An introductory letter should also explain what is involved and the likely duration of the interview and should give assurances about confidentiality. Interviews should always be conducted at interviewees' convenience, which for people who work during the day will often be in the evening. The setting of an interview affects the content, and it is usually preferable to interview people in their own homes.

Conclusion

Qualitative interviewing is a flexible and powerful tool that can open up many new areas for research. It is worth remembering that answers to interview questions about behaviour will not necessarily correspond with observational studies: what people say they do is not always the same as what they can be observed doing. That said, qualitative interviews can be used to enable practising clinicians to investigate research questions of immediate relevance to their everyday work, which would otherwise be difficult to investigate. Few researchers would consider embarking on a new research technique without some form of training, and training in research interviewing skills is available from universities and specialist research organisations.

Further reading

Fontana A, Frey JH. Interviewing: the art of science. In: Denzin NK, Lincoln YS, eds. *Handbook of qualitative research*. London: Sage, 1994:361–76.

Kvale S. *InterViews: an introduction to qualitative research interviewing*. London: Sage, 1996.

References

1 Britten N. Patients' ideas about medicines: a qualitative study in a general practice population. *British Journal of General Practice* 1994;**44**:465–8.
2 Black N, Thompson E. Obstacles to medical audit: British doctors speak. *Social Science and Medicine* 1993;**36**:849–56.
3 Gantley M, Davis DP, Murcott A. Sudden infant death syndrome: links with infant care practices. *Br Med J* 1993;**306**:16–20.
4 Green JM. The views of single-handed general practitioners: a qualitative study. *Br Med J* 1993;**307**:607–10.
5 Britten N. Hospital consultants' views of their patients. *Sociology of Health and Illness* 1991;**13**:83–97.
6 Bradley CP. Uncomfortable prescribing decisions: a critical incident study. *Br Med J* 1992;**304**:294–6.
7 Patton MQ. *How to use qualitative methods in evaluation*. London: Sage, 1987:108–43.
8 Cannon S. Social research in stressful settings: difficulties for the sociologist studying the treatment of breast cancer. *Sociology of Health and Illness* 1989;**11**:62–77.
9 Oakley A. Interviewing women: a contradiction in terms. In: Roberts H, ed. *Doing feminist research*. London: Routledge and Kegan Paul, 1981:30–61.
10 Whyte WF. Interviewing in field research. In: Burgess RG, ed. *Field research: a sourcebook and field manual*. London: George Allen and Unwin, 1982:111–22.
11 Holstein JA, Gubrium JF. *The active interview*. London: Sage, 1995:56.
12 Field PA, Morse JM. *Nursing research: the application of qualitative approaches*. London: Chapman & Hall, 1989.
13 Mays N, Pope C. Rigour and qualitative research. *Br Med J* 1995;**311**:109–112.
14 Holland J, Ramazanoglu C, Scott S, Sharpe S, Thomson R. Sex, gender and power: young women's sexuality in the shadow of AIDS. *Sociology of Health and Illness* 1990;**12**:36–50.

3 Focus groups with users and providers of health care

JENNY KITZINGER

What are focus groups?

Focus groups are a form of group interview that capitalises on communication between research participants in order to generate data. Although group interviews are often employed simply as a quick and convenient way to collect data from several people simultaneously, focus groups explicitly use group interaction to provide distinctive types of data. This means that instead of the researcher asking each person to respond to a question in turn, people are encouraged to talk to one another, asking questions, exchanging anecdotes and commenting on each others' experiences and points of view (see Box 1).[1]

Focus groups were originally employed in communication studies to explore the effects of films and television programmes.[2] Not surprisingly, given their history, focus groups are a popular method for assessing health education messages and examining public understandings of illness and of health behaviours.[3-7] They have also become widely used to examine people's experiences of disease and of health services.[8,9] In addition, the method has proved to be an effective technique for exploring the attitudes and needs of staff.[10,11] For example, focus groups have been used to examine people's attitudes toward smoking,[12] the health needs of lesbians,[13] ethnic minority views on screening procedures,[14] the impact of AIDS health education information,[15] the experience of breast cancer[16] and professional responses to changing management arrangements for community nurses.[17]

Box 1—Interaction between participants can be used:

* to highlight the respondents' attitudes, priorities, language and framework of understanding
* to encourage research participants to generate and explore their own questions and to develop their own analysis of common experiences
* to encourage a variety of communication from participants – tapping into a wide range and different forms of discourse
* to help to identify group norms/cultural values
* to provide insight into the operation of group social processes in the articulation of knowledge (e.g. through the examination of what information is sensitive within the group)
* to encourage open conversation about embarrassing subjects and to permit the expression of criticism;
* generally to facilitate the expression of ideas and experiences that might be left underdeveloped in an interview and to illuminate the research participants' perspectives through the debate within the group.

The idea behind the focus group method is that group processes can help people to explore and clarify their views in ways that would be less easily accessible in a one-to-one interview. Group discussion is particularly appropriate when the interviewer has a series of open-ended questions and wishes to encourage research participants to explore the issues of importance to them, in their own vocabulary, generating their own questions and pursuing their own priorities. When group dynamics work well the co-participants act as co-researchers, taking the research in new and often unexpected directions.

Group work also helps researchers tap into the many different forms of communication that people use in day-to-day interaction, including jokes, anecdotes, teasing and arguing. Gaining access to such a variety of communication is useful because people's knowledge and attitudes are not entirely encapsulated in reasoned responses to direct questions. Everyday forms of communication may tell us as much, if not more, about what people know or experience. In this sense, focus groups "reach the parts that other methods cannot reach", revealing dimensions of understanding that often remain untapped by more conventional data collection techniques.

Tapping into such inter-personal communication is also important because it can highlight (sub)cultural values or group norms. Through analysing the operation or humour, consensus and dissent and examining different types of narrative employed within the group, the researcher can identify shared and common knowledge.[18] This makes focus groups a particularly culturally sensitive data collection technique, which is why it is so often employed in cross-cultural research and work with ethnic minorities. It also makes focus groups useful in studies examining why different sections of the population make differential use of health services.[19] For similar reasons, focus groups are useful for studying dominant cultural values (for example, exposing dominant narratives about sexuality)[20] and for examining work place cultures – the ways in which, for example, staff cope with working with terminally ill patients or deal with the stresses of an Accident and Emergency department.

The presence of other research participants can compromise the usual confidentiality of a research setting, so special care should be taken, especially when working with "captive" populations (such as patients in a hospice, or patients attending a clinic). However, it should not be assumed that groups are always more inhibiting than the supposed privacy of a one-to-one interview or that focus groups are inappropriate when researching sensitive topics. In fact, quite the opposite may be true. Group work can actively facilitate the discussion of taboo topics because the less inhibited members of the group break the ice for shyer participants.[13] Co-participants can also provide mutual support in expressing feelings that are common to their group, but which they consider to deviate from mainstream culture (or the assumed culture of the researcher). This is particularly important when researching stigmatised or taboo experiences (for example, bereavement or sexual violence).

Focus group methods are also popular with those conducting *action research* (see Chapter 7) and those concerned to empower research participants, who can become an active part of the research development and analysis process.[21] Group participants may develop particular perspectives as a consequence of talking with other people who have similar experiences. For example, group dynamics can allow for a shift from personal self-blaming psychological explanations ("I'm stupid not to have understood what the doctor was telling me" or "I should have been stronger – I should have asked the right questions,") to the exploration of structural solutions ("If we've all felt confused about what we've been told maybe having a leaflet would help" or "What about being able to take away a tape-recording of the consultation?").

Some researchers have also noted that group discussions can generate more critical comments than interviews.[22] For example, Geis and his colleagues, in their study of the lovers of people with AIDS, found that there were more angry comments about the medical community in the group discussions than in the individual interviews: ". . . perhaps the synergism of the group 'kept the anger going' and allowed each participant to reinforce another's vented feelings of frustration and rage. . ."[23] Using a method that facilitates the expression of criticism and, at the same time, the exploration of different types of solutions, is invaluable if one is seeking to improve services. Such a method is especially appropriate when working with particularly disempowered patient populations who are often reluctant to give negative feedback or may feel that any problems result from their own inadequacies.[24]

Conducting a focus group study

Sampling and group composition

Focus group studies can consist of anything from half a dozen to over 50 groups, depending on the aims of the project and the resources available. Even just a few groups can generate a large amount of data, and for this reason many studies using focus groups rely on a modest number of groups. Some studies combine this method with other data collection techniques; for example focus group discussion of a questionnaire is an ideal way of testing out the phrasing of questions for a survey and is also useful when seeking to explain or explore survey results.[25,26]

Although it may be possible to work with a representative sample of a small population, most focus group studies use *theoretical sampling* whereby participants are selected to reflect a range of the total study population or to test particular hypotheses. Imaginative sampling is crucial. Most people now recognise class or ethnicity as important sampling variables. However, it is also worth considering other variables. For example, when exploring women's experiences of maternity care it may be advisable explicitly to include groups of women who were sexually abused as children as they can provide unique insights about respectful care or the power relationships underlying the delivery of care.[27]

Most researchers recommend aiming for homogeneity within each group in order to capitalise on people's shared experiences. However, it can also be advantageous on occasions to bring together a diverse group (for example, from a range of professions) in order to maximise exploration of different perspectives within a group setting. However, it is important to be aware of how hierarchy within the group may affect the data. A nursing auxiliary is likely to be inhibited by the presence of a consultant from the same hospital, for example.

The groups can be "naturally occurring", such as people who work together, or may be drawn together specifically for the research. By using pre-existing groups, one is able to observe fragments of interactions that approximate to naturally occurring data (such as might have been collected by participant observation). An additional advantage is that friends and colleagues can relate each other's comments to actual incidents in their shared daily lives. They may challenge each other on contradictions between what they profess to believe and how they actually behave (for example, "how about that time you didn't use a glove while taking blood from a patient?").

It would be naïve, however, to assume that group data are by definition "natural" in the sense that such interactions would have occurred without the group being convened for this purpose. Rather than assuming that sessions inevitably reflect everyday interactions (although sometimes they will), the group should be used to encourage people to engage with one another, formulate their ideas and draw out cognitive structures that have not been articulated previously.

Finally, it is important to consider the appropriateness of group work for different study populations and to think about how to overcome potential difficulties. Group work can facilitate collecting information from people who cannot read or write. The "safety in numbers" factor may also encourage the participation of those who are wary of an interviewer or those who are anxious about talking.[28] However, group work can compound difficulties in communication if each person has a different disability. In a study assessing residential care for the elderly, I conducted a focus group that included one person who had impaired hearing, another with senile dementia and a third with partial paralysis affecting her speech. This severely restricted interaction between research participants and confirmed some of the staff's predictions about the limitations of group work with this population. However, such problems could be resolved by thinking more carefully about the composition of the group and sometimes group participants could help to translate for each other. It should also be noted that some of the old people who might have been unable to sustain a one-to-one interview were able to take part in the group, contributing intermittently. Even some residents whom staff had suggested should be excluded from the research because they were "unresponsive" eventually responded to the lively conversations generated by their co-residents and were able to contribute their point of view (see Box 2). Considerations of communication difficulties should not rule out group work, but must be considered as a factor.

Box 2—Some potential sampling advantages in the use of focus groups

- Does not discriminate against people who cannot read or write
- Can encourage participation from those who are reluctant to be interviewed on their own (such as those intimidated by the formality and isolation of a one-to-one interview)
- Can encourage contributions from people who feel they have nothing to say or who are deemed "unresponsive patients" (but who engage in the discussion generated by other group members).

Running the groups

Sessions should be relaxed: a comfortable setting, refreshments and sitting round in a circle will help to establish the right atmosphere. The ideal group size is from four to eight people. Sessions may last around one or two hours (or extend into a whole afternoon or a series of meetings). The group facilitator should explain that the aim of focus groups is to encourage people to talk to each other rather than to address themselves to the researcher. She/he may take a back seat at first, allowing for a type of "structured eavesdropping".[29] Later on in the session, however, the facilitator can adopt a more interventionist style, urging debate to continue beyond the stage at which it might otherwise have ended and encouraging members of the group to discuss the inconsistencies both between participants and within their own thinking.

The facilitator may sometimes take on a "devil's advocate" role in order to provoke debate.[30] Disagreements within groups can be used to encourage participants to elucidate their point of view and to clarify why they think as they do. Differences between individual one-off interviews have to be analysed by the researchers through armchair theorising after the event; differences between members of focus groups should be explored in situ with the help of the research participants.

The facilitator may also take materials along to the group to help to focus and provoke debate.[31] For example, I often present research participants with pictures from the mass media, or advertisements (with their strap lines removed).[32] Other people take in objects. For example, Chui and Knight passed around a speculum during their group discussions about cervical smears,[14] and in Wilkinson's study of breast cancer one woman spontaneously pulled out and passed around her prosthesis. Such opportunities to see and handle objects not usually available provoked considerable discussion and provided important insights.[16]

An alternative or additional type of prompt involves presenting the group with a series of statements on large cards. The group members are asked collectively to sort these cards into different piles depending on, for example, their degree of agreement or disagreement with that point of view or the importance they assign to that particular aspect of service. For example, I have used such cards to explore public understandings of HIV transmission (placing statements about "types" of people into different risk categories), old people's experiences of residential care (assigning degrees of importance to different statements about the quality of their care), and midwives' views of their professional responsibilities (placing a series of statements about midwives' roles along an agree–disagree continuum). Exercises such as these encourage participants to concentrate on one another (rather than on the group facilitator) and force them to explain their different perspectives. The final layout of the cards is less important than the discussion that it generates. Facilitators may also use this kind of exercise as a way of checking out their own assessment of what has emerged from the group. In this case, it is best to take along a series of blank cards and only fill them out toward the end of the session, using statements generated during the course of the discussion. Finally, it may be beneficial to present research participants with a brief questionnaire, or the opportunity to speak to the facilitator privately, giving each member of the group the opportunity to record private comments after the group session has been completed.

Ideally the group's discussions should be tape recorded and transcribed. If this is not possible, then it is vital to take careful notes, and researchers may find it useful to involve the group in recording key issues on a flip chart.

Analysis and writing up

The process of analysing qualitative data is discussed in the penultimate chapter of this book. Here I simply wish to note that in analysing focus groups it is important to take full advantage and cognisance of the interaction between research participants. For discussion of different ways of working with focus group data, including using computer assisted packages, conversational or discourse analysis, or examining "sensitive moments" in group interaction see Frankland and Bloor,[12] Myers and Macnaghten[33] and Kitzinger and Farquhar.[34]

Conclusion

To sum up, this chapter has introduced some of the factors to consider when designing or evaluating a focus group study. In particular, it has drawn attention to the overt exploitation and exploration of interactions in focus group discussion. Group data are neither more nor less authentic than data collected by other methods; rather focus groups may be the most appropriate method for researching particular types of question. Direct observation may be more appropriate for studies of social roles and formal organisations, but focus groups are particularly suited to the study of attitudes and experiences. Interviews may be more appropriate for tapping into individual biographies, but focus groups are more suitable for examining how knowledge and, more importantly, ideas develop, operate and are expressed within a given cultural context. Questionnaires are more appropriate for obtaining quantitative information and explaining how many people hold a certain (pre-defined) opinion. However, focus groups are better for exploring exactly how those opinions are constructed or, depending on your theoretical background, how different "discourses" are expressed and mobilised. (Indeed, discourse analysis of focus group data can challenge the idea that "opinions" exist at all as predefined entities to be "discovered" within individuals).[35]

Focus groups are not an easy option. The data they generate can be both cumbersome and complex. Yet the method is basically straightforward and need not be intimidating for either the researcher or the participants. Perhaps the very best way of working out whether focus groups might be appropriate in any particular study is to read a selection of other people's focus groups reports and then to try out a few pilot groups with friends or acquaintances.

Further reading

Barbour R, Kitzinger J. *Developing focus group research: politics, theory and practice.* London: Sage, 1999.

References

1 Kitzinger J. The methodology of focus groups: the importance of interactions between research participants. *Sociology of Health and Illness* 1994;**16**:103–21.
2 Merton RK. *The focused interview.* Glencoe, IL: Free Press, 1956.
3 Basch C. Focus group interview: an under-utilised research technique for improving theory and practice in health education. *Health Education Quarterly* 1987;**14**:411–48.
4 Ritchie JE, Herscovitch F, Norfor JB. Beliefs of blue collar workers regarding coronary risk behaviours. *Health Education Research* 1994;**9**:95–103.
5 Duke SS, Gordon-Sosby K, Reynolds KD, Gram, IT. A study of breast cancer detection practices and beliefs in black women attending public health clinics. *Health Education Research* 1994;**9**:331–42.
6 Khan M, Manderson L. Focus groups in tropical diseases research. *Health Policy and Planning* 1992;**7**:56–66.
7 Morgan D. *Focus groups as qualitative research.* London: Sage, 1988.
8 Murray S, Tapson J, Turnbull L, McCallum J, Little A. Listening to local voices: adapting rapid appraisal to assess health and social needs in general practice. *Br Med J* 1994;**308**:698–700.
9 Gregory S, McKie L. The smear test: listening to women's views. *Nursing Standard* 1991;**5**:32–6.
10 Brown J, Lent B, Sas G. Identifying and treating wife abuse. *Journal of Family Practice* 1993;**36**:185–91.
11 Denning JD, Verschelden C. Using the focus group in assessing training needs: empowering child welfare workers. *Child Welfare League of America* 1993;**72**(6):569–79.
12 Frankland C, Bloor M. Some issues arising in the systematic analysis of focus group materials. In: Barbour R, Kitzinger J. *Developing focus group research: politics, theory and practice.* London: Sage, 1999.
13 Farquhar C. Are focus groups suitable for 'sensitive' topics? In: Barbour R, Kitzinger J. *Developing focus group research: politics, theory and practice.* London: Sage, 1999.
14 Chui L, Knight, D. How useful are focus groups for obtaining the views of minority groups? In: Barbour R, Kitzinger J. *Developing focus group research: politics, theory and practice.* London: Sage, 1999.

15 Kitzinger J. Understanding AIDS: researching audience perceptions of Acquired Immune Deficiency Syndrome. In: Eldridge J. ed. *Getting the Message; news, truth and power.* London: Routledge, 1993:271–305.

16 Wilkinson S. Focus groups in health research. *Journal of Health Psychology* 1998;**3**:323–42.

17 Barbour R. Are focus groups an appropriate tool for studying organisational change? In: Barbour R, Kitzinger J. *Developing focus group research: politics, theory and practice.* London: Sage, 1999.

18 Hughes D, Dumont K. Using focus groups to facilitate culturally anchored research. *American Journal of Community Psychology* 1993;**21**:775–806.

19 Naish J, Brown J, Denton, B. Intercultural consultations: investigation of factors that deter non-English speaking women from attending their general practitioners for cervical screening. *Br Med J* 1994;**309**:1126–8.

20 Barker G, Rich S. Influences on adolescent sexuality in Nigeria and Kenya: findings from recent focus-group discussions. *Studies in Family Planning* 1992;**23**:199–210.

21 Baker R, Hinton R. Do focus groups facilitate meaningful participation in social research? In: Barbour R, Kitzinger J. *Developing focus group research: politics, theory and practice.* London: Sage, 1999.

22 Watts M, Ebbutt D. More than the sum of the parts: research methods in group interviewing. *British Educational Research Journal* 1987;**13**:25–34.

23 Geis S, Fuller R, Rush J. Lovers of AIDS victims: psychosocial stresses and counselling needs. *Death Studies* 1986;**10**:43–53.

24 DiMatteo M, Kahn K, Berry S. Narratives of birth and the postpartum: an analysis of the focus group responses of new mothers. *Birth* 1993;**20**:204.

25 Kitzinger J. Focus groups: method or madness? In: Boulton M. ed. *Challenge and innovation: methodological advances in social research on HIV/AIDS.* London: Taylor & Francis, 1994:159–75.

26 O'Brien K. Improving survey questionnaires through focus groups. In Morgan D. ed. *Successful focus groups: advancing the state of the art.* London: Sage, 1993:105–18.

27 Kitzinger J. Recalling the pain: incest survivors' experiences of obstetrics and gynaecology. *Nursing Times* 1990;**86**:38–40.

28 Lederman L. High apprehensives talk about communication apprehension and its effects on their behaviour. *Communication Quarterly* 1983;**31**:233–7.

29 Powney J. Structured eavesdropping. *Research Intelligence (Journal of the British Educational Research Foundation)* 1988;**28**:3–4.

30 MacDougall C, Baum F. The devil's advocate: a strategy to avoid groupthink and stimulate discussion in focus groups. *Qualitative Health Research* 1997;**7**:532–41.

31 Morgan D, Kreguer R. *The focus group kit* volumes 1-6. London: Sage, 1997.

32 Kitzinger J. Audience understanding AIDS: a discussion of methods. *Sociology of Health and Illness* 1990;**12**:319–35.

33 Myers G, Macnaghten P. Can focus groups be analyzed as talk? In: Barbour R, Kitzinger J. *Developing focus group research: politics, theory and practice.* London: Sage, 1999.

34 Kitzinger J, Farquhar C. The analytical potential of 'sensitive moments' in focus group discussions. In: Barbour R, Kitzinger J. *Developing focus group research: politics, theory and practice.* London: Sage, 1999.

35 Waterton C, Wynne B. Can focus groups access community views? In: Barbour R, Kitzinger J. *Developing focus group research: politics, theory and practice.* London: Sage, 1999.

4 Observational methods in health care settings

CATHERINE POPE, NICHOLAS MAYS

Chapters 2 and 3 have described two methods that allow researchers to collect data on what people say. Interviewees and focus group members report their beliefs and attitudes, and they may also talk about their actions and behaviour. One benefit of these methods is that they provide a relatively quick way of gathering this sort of information. However, we cannot be sure that what people say they do is what they really do.[1,2] Observational methods go some way towards addressing this problem – instead of asking questions about behaviour, the researcher systematically watches people and events to observe people's everyday behaviours and interactions.

It can be argued that observation is the basis of all scientific inquiry. It is the building block of the natural sciences: the biologist observes development of cell structures and the chemist observes the changes that occur in chemical reactions. Observational studies of populations or communities are used in epidemiology to look for patterns in the incidence of disease, thereby suggesting possible causes. At the individual level, research in clinical and experimental psychology also relies on observation, as does the monitoring of a patient in a hospital bed.

Qualitative observational methods differ from these types of observation. Observation in the social sciences involves the systematic, detailed observation of behaviour and talk. One of the crucial differences between this type of observation and that conducted in the natural sciences is that in the social world those we observe can use language to describe, reflect on, and argue about what they are doing. This shared language and understanding of the social world makes social science research very different from the observation of laboratory rats or electrons. Unlike the natural sciences, it tends to be *naturalistic* in that people are studied in situ with minimal interference by the researcher.[3]

Observational techniques are most frequently employed in the branch of social science known as *ethnography* (literally, "the study of the people"). The premise underlying ethnography is that in order to understand a group of people, the researcher needs to observe their daily lives, ideally living with, and living like them. As Goffman put it, to "submit oneself in the company of the members to the daily round of petty contingencies to which they are subject".[4] Ethnography emphasises the importance of understanding the symbolic world in which people live, seeing things the way they do and grasping the meanings they draw on to make sense of their experiences. To do this, ethnographers work in the same way as the anthropologists who study remote tribes or cultures, learning to understand the language, concepts, and practices of the group being studied.

Ethnographic research often combines observational methods with analysis of data from other sources, such as documents or interviews, but observational methods can be used exclusively. While this chapter is concerned primarily with observational methods used in qualitative research, many of the examples provided come from ethnographic studies of health and health services that have used observation alongside other research methods.

Observational methods in health and health services research

One major influence on ethnography was the so called "Chicago School" of sociology, whose members systematically observed the lives of different, often marginal or deviant social groups in that city such as gamblers, crooks, drug addicts and jazz musicians from the 1920s onwards. Early examples of the use of observational methods in health and health services research tended to mimic the ethnographic model of the Chicago School. For example, Roth's pioneering study of a TB sanatorium developed the concept of the "patient career" – a series of stages that the patient passes through during treatment – and the idea of "timetables" that structure the treatment process for both patients and staff.[5] In the UK, there have been a number of observational studies of accident and emergency (A and E) departments. Jeffery documented the categorisation by staff of patients into the "good" and the "rubbish", the latter consisting of drunks, tramps, para-suicides and other patients who, because of the conflicting demands and pressures on staff, were seen as inappropriate attenders at A and E.[6] Dingwall and Murray developed and extended this model using observation and interviews to examine how children were managed in A and E.[7] In another study, Hughes observed reception clerks' use of discretion when prioritising and categorising A and E attenders.[8] These studies provide clear insights as to how and why patients are managed as they are in such settings. The behaviour of staff in categorising and labelling patients was so embedded in the organisational culture that only an outsider would have considered it noteworthy. It is unlikely that interviews alone would have uncovered the patient typologies used by staff and the different patterns of care they provoked.

Other observational research has been used to develop explanations for relationships or associations found in quantitative work. Bloor's observational study of ear, nose and throat (ENT) surgeons was designed to complement a statistical analysis of variations between areas and surgeons in rates for childhood tonsillectomy.[9] Bloor systematically analysed how surgeons made their decisions to operate and discovered that individual doctors had different "rules of thumb" for deciding whether or not to operate. While one surgeon might take clinical signs as the chief indication for surgery, another might be prepared to operate in the absence of such indications at the time of consultation if there was evidence that repeated episodes of tonsillitis were affecting a child's education. More recently, Hughes and Griffiths observed cardiac catheterisation clinics and neurological admissions conferences to explore how decisions about priorities were made when resources were constrained.[10] They showed that patient selection differs dramatically between the two specialties and suggested that this can be explained by the way rationing decisions are made in each. They showed that in cardiology, decisions tend be framed around the idea of poor prognosis or unsuitability of the patient – "ruling out" – whereas in neurology, greater weight tends to be placed on "ruling in" – identifying factors that might make an individual patient especially deserving of help. These analyses begin to explain why different types of patients come to be treated and might be helpful in designing more explicit priority-setting systems in future, which are, nonetheless, rooted in clinical routines.

Alongside research on the everyday work of health professionals,[11-13] observational methods have been used to look at other, crucial members of the health care team – for example, the clerks who deal with inpatient waiting lists.[14] This research, based on extended periods spent observing the admissions office in a district hospital, uncovered how surgical and administrative preferences dictated how and when patients were selected from surgical waiting lists. It demonstrated that waiting lists did not operate as a queue, following the rule of "first come, first served"; rather different admission decisions were informed by such things as the sorts of cases needed for teaching medical students, or the ease with which patients could be contacted. The notion of a "store" of patients from which staff constructed operating lists (rather than a simple queue) derived from this research, has major implications for the design of effective policies aimed at reducing waiting times.

There is also a growing body of more explicitly policy-oriented observational research. Strong and Robinson's analysis of the introduction of general management in the NHS in the mid 1980s involved the researchers sitting in on management meetings and conducting lengthy interviews with those involved in the transition to the new-look NHS following the Griffiths Report.[15] More recently, under the auspices of the Economic and Social Research Council's Contracts and Competition programme, observational methods were used to look at the relative importance of relations built on trust versus more adversarial relationships in negotiating effective contracts for health services in the internal market of the first half of the 1990s.[16]

Using observational methods: access to the field and research roles

The first task in observational research is choosing and gaining access to the setting or "field". Occasionally, access to the setting leads to opportunistic research – Roth happened to have TB when he conducted his research on life in a TB hospital – but few researchers have it this easy (or difficult). Most have to decide on the type of setting they are interested in and negotiate access. The choice or sampling of a setting is typically *purposive*, as in most qualitative research. The idea is not to choose a setting in order to generalise to a whole population (as would be the case in a statistical sample), but to select a group or setting, usually informed by prior knowledge and theoretical work, which is likely to demonstrate salient features and events or categories of behaviour relevant to the research question. Hughes and Griffiths deliberately selected the very different settings of a neurology and a cardiology clinic as the basis for their research on micro-level rationing to allow them to look at two contrasting areas of clinical practice where significant resource constraints apply.

Access to a setting or group is usually negotiated via a "gatekeeper", someone in a position to allow and, often, to facilitate the research. In medical settings, this may involve negotiating with several different staff, including doctors, nurses, managers or members of hospital boards. This first point of contact is important: she or he may be seen to sponsor or support the research and this can affect how the researcher is perceived by the group. Once "inside", in the initial phases of the research, there may be problems striking up sufficient rapport and empathy with the group to enable the research to be conducted. The researcher may be expected to reciprocate the favour of having been granted access. It is not uncommon for observers to become embroiled in the life of the ward, clinic or the general practice, to the extent of being asked to assist with clerking patients, running errands, or simply holding a nervous patient's hand.

It is important to consider the characteristics of the researcher as well as those of the group or setting, as this too influences the process of data collection: being male or female, young or old, naïve or experienced, can affect the interactions between the researcher and the researched.[17–19] Once accepted by the group, there is the problem of avoiding "going native", that is becoming so immersed in the group culture that the researcher either loses the ability to stand back and analyse the setting, or finds it extremely difficult or emotionally draining to conclude the data collection.

The observer may adopt different roles according to the type of setting and to how access was obtained. Some health care settings, such as the A and E department, are semi-public spaces, and it may be possible to adhere closely to the role of detached observer, unobtrusively watching what goes on. However, the presence of an observer, particularly in more private settings, may stimulate modifications in behaviour or action – the so-called Hawthorne effect[20,21] – although this effect seems to reduce over time. Those being observed may also begin to reflect on their activities and question the observer about what they are doing.

The impact of the observer on the setting can be minimised by participating in the activities taking place while observing them. Sometimes this is done covertly, as in Goffman's research on the asylum where he worked as physical education instructor, or in Rosenhan's study[22] where observers feigned psychiatric symptoms to gain admittance to a psychiatric hospital. There are important ethical issues in such research – notably that of informed consent. Covert research roles may be justified in certain circumstances such as researching particularly sensitive topics or difficult-to-access groups. Most research in health care settings is overt, although the extent to which all members of the group know about the research may vary. For example, staff and patients (and sometimes staff but not patients) may be aware that observation is taking place, but they may not know the specific research questions or areas of interest. Dingwall has suggested that such research often entails continual, informal negotiation of access and consent, although he concedes that this may not be feasible or practical in all settings.[23]

Recording observational data

Observational research relies on the researcher acting as the research instrument and document the world she or he observes. This requires not only good observational skills, but good memory and clear, detailed and systematic recording. The research role adopted, whether covert or overt, participant or non-participant, can influence the process of recording. Sometimes it is possible to take notes or record information in the setting, at others times this may be impractical or off-putting. Remembering events and conversations is crucial, and is a skill that requires practice. Memory can be aided by the use of jotted notes made where possible during observation (one way of making such notes is to find excuses to leave the setting for a few minutes to write up – frequent trips to the lavatory are often used for this). These notes record key events, timings, quotes or actions. The recording of observational material can be structured around a list of items to observe and describe, for example, the layout of the setting, the character of each participant, or a specific set of activities.

Silverman used such an approach in his study of paediatric cardiology clinics. Having observed ten clinics, he developed a coding form for recording "disposal" decisions, which covered the factors that appeared, on the basis of these initial observations, to be involved in those decisions – things such as clinical and social factors, and how and when decisions were communicated to patients.[24]

Another approach is to focus on "critical incidents" – discrete events or specific contexts – and to describe and document these separately.[25] However they are taken, it is essential that field notes are written up in full as soon as possible afterwards. These are detailed, highly descriptive accounts of what was observed, which provide a chronological account of the events, and a description of the people involved, their talk and their behaviour. It is important that concrete descriptions are recorded, and not simply impressions. Accordingly, there are conventions for denoting different types of observation, such as verbatim quotes from conversations, non-verbal behaviour and gestures or spatial representations. In addition, the researcher needs to document his or her personal impressions, feelings and reactions to these observations. These more reflexive data are typically recorded separately in a field diary documenting the progress of the research.

In observational research, is it important to consider the representativeness of periods spent in the chosen setting. It is seldom possible or feasible to observe the setting "round the clock", but it is important to spend as much time as possible with the group being studied to ensure adequate coverage of different time periods. This may mean making sure that data are collected on different days or at different times. Some researchers choose to sample random blocks of time, or observe particular aspects of the setting, or particular individuals for a fixed period and then move on – say, observing the clinic from the reception area then moving to the nurses' station. It is a mistake to think that the observer will necessarily capture "everything". Even the using of several observers, or video/audio taping cannot ensure this. The combination of the practicalities of observation, recall and perception means that it is simply not possible to remember or record everything. Nonetheless, as far as possible, the researcher's task is to document in detail what happened.

This descriptive raw material cannot and does not provide explanations – it is the researcher's task to sift, decode and make sense of the data. This analytical process usually begins during the data collection phase of the research: in the example of Silverman's study, ideas about the initial data informed the development of the coding sheet.[24] Emerging categories or tentative hypotheses about the data may be tested during the fieldwork; more cases or examples (or contradictory ones), may be sought.

Theorising from observational research

The analysis of observational data is described in more detail in Chapter 8. In essence it entails some form of *content analysis*, and an iterative process of developing categories from the field notes and testing and refining them to develop theories and explanatory models. Different methodological and theoretical perspectives can influence this analytical process and the way in which observational data are treated. These different stances are complex and hotly debated, and there is insufficient space to describe them in detail here; interested readers may wish to consult the references supplied.[26-28]

Quality in observational studies

Observational research relies on the researcher to act directly as the research instrument. The quality of observational studies depends more than most methods on the quality of the researcher. This places a particular responsibility on the researcher to provide detailed descriptions of data collection and analysis. Details about how the research was conducted are crucial to assessing its integrity, for example, enabling the reader to know how much time was spent in the field, the researcher's proximity to the action or behaviour, how typical the events recorded were and whether any attempts were made to verify the observations made (such as observing comparable settings or seeking out other sources of information, such as documents). It may be possible to check the verisimilitude (the appearance of truthfulness) of an observational study against previous research in similar settings or with similar groups, but perhaps the ultimate test for observational research, is *congruence*:[29] how far the research provides the necessary instructions or rules which might enable another researcher to enter and pass in that setting or group.

Chapter 8 revisits some of these issues concerning quality in qualitative research. Done well, that is systematically and carefully, observational studies can reveal and explain important features of life in health care settings. The very best, like Goffman's classic study of the Asylum,[4] can generate insightful and enduring concepts that can be applied to other settings and that add to our knowledge of the social world.

Further reading

Strong P. *The ceremonial order of the clinic*. London: Routledge, 1979.
Becker HS, Geer B. Participant observation: the analysis of qualitative field data. In: Burgess RG. ed. *Field Research: a source book and field manual*. London: Allen and Unwin, 1982: 239–50.

References

1 Silverman D. *Interpreting qualitative data*. London: Sage, 1994.
2 Heritage J. *Garfinkel and Ethnomethodology*. Cambridge: Polity, 1984.
3 Blumer H. *Symbolic interactionism*. Engelwood Cliffs, NJ: Prentice Hall, 1969.
4 Goffman E. *Asylums: essays on the social situation of mental patients and other inmates*. Harmondsworth: Penguin, 1961.
5 Roth J. *Timetables*. New York: Bobbs-Merrill, 1963.
6 Jeffery R. Normal rubbish: deviant patients in casualty departments. *Sociology of Health and Illness* 1979;**1**:90–108.
7 Dingwall R, Murray T. Categorisation in accident departments: 'good' patients, 'bad' patients and children. *Sociology of Health and Illness* 1983;**5**:127–48.
8 Hughes D. Paper and people: the work of the casualty reception clerk. *Sociology of Health and Illness* 1989;**11**:382–408.
9 Bloor M. Bishop Berkeley and the adenotonsillectomy enigma: an exploration of the social construction of medical disposals. *Sociology* 1976;**10**:43–61.
10 Hughes D, Griffiths L. 'Ruling in' and 'ruling out': two approaches to the micro-rationing of health care. *Social Science and Medicine* 1997;**44**:589–99.
11 Clarke P, Bowling A. Quality of life in long stay institutions for the elderly: an observational study of long stay hospital and nursing home care. *Social Science and Medicine* 1990;**30**:1201–10.
12 Atkinson P. *Medical talk and medical work*. London: Sage, 1995.
13 Fox N. *The social meaning of surgery*. Milton Keynes: Open University Press, 1988.
14 Pope C. Trouble in store: some thoughts on the management of waiting lists. *Sociology of Health and Illness* 1991;**13**:193–212.
15 Strong P, Robinson J. *The NHS: under new management*. Milton Keynes: Open University Press, 1990.
16 Flynn R, Williams G, Pickard S. *Markets and networks: contracting in community health services*. Buckingham: Open University Press, 1996.
17 Warren C, Rasmussen P. Sex and gender in field research. *Urban Life* 1977;**6**:349–69.
18 Aldridge A. Negotiating status: social scientists and the Anglican clergy. In: Hertz R, Imber J. eds. *Studying elites using qualitative methods*. London: Sage, 1995.
19 Ostrander S. 'Surely you're not just in this to be helpful': access, rapport, and interviews in three studies of elites. In: Hertz R, Imber J. eds. *Studying elites using qualitative methods*. London: Sage, 1995.

20 Roethlisberger FJ, Dickson WJ. *Management and the worker.* Cambridge, MA: Harvard University Press, 1939.
21 Holden J and Bower P. How does misuse of the term 'Hawthorne effect' affect the interpretation of research outcomes? (Questions and Answers) *Journal of Health Services Research and Policy* 1998;3:192.
22 Rosenhan DL. On being sane in insane places. *Science* 1973;**179**:250–8.
23 Dingwall R. Ethics and ethnography. *Sociological Review* 1980;**28**:871–91.
24 Silverman D. The child as a social object: Down's Syndrome children in a paediatric cardiology clinic. *Sociology of Health and Illness* 1989;3:254–74.
25 Erlandson D, Harris E, Skipper B, Allen S. *Doing naturalistic inquiry: a guide to methods.* Newbury Park, CA: Sage, 1993.
26 Van Maanan J. *Tales of the field: on writing ethnography.* Chicago: University of Chicago Press, 1988.
27 Hammersley M. *The dilemma of qualitative method: Herbert Blumer and the Chicago Tradition.* London: Routledge, 1989.
28 Feldman M. *Strategies for interpreting qualitative data* Qualitative Research Methods 33. Newbury Park, CA: Sage, 1995.
29 Fielding N. *Researching social life.* London: Sage, 1993.

5 Using the Delphi and nominal group technique in health services research

JEREMY JONES, DUNCAN HUNTER

What are consensus methods?

Quantitative methods such as meta-analysis have been developed to provide statistical overviews of the results of clinical trials, and to resolve inconsistencies between the results of different published studies. Where unanimity of opinion does not exist due to a lack of scientific evidence, as well as where there is contradictory evidence on an issue, consensus methods can also be used. They attempt both to assess the extent of agreement (consensus measurement) as well as resolve disagreement (consensus development), and generally consider evidence from a wider range of study types than is the case in statistical reviews. Such methods allow a greater role for the qualitative assessment of evidence, though they are often concerned with deriving quantitative estimates from the evidence (for example, estimating probabilities for decision analysis or cost-effectiveness analysis).

The three formal consensus methods most commonly used in health services research are:

- the Delphi process
- the nominal group technique (NGT) also known as the expert panel
- the consensus development conference (not considered in this chapter).

The Delphi method and NGT seek to maximise the benefits from having informed panels consider a problem (often termed "process gain") while minimising the disadvantages associated with collective decision-making ("process loss"). Typically, group decision-making is dominated by one individual or by coalitions representing vested interests, with individuals often being unready to retract long-held and publicly stated opinions in open meetings. Formal consensus methods are structured to avoid these drawbacks and to use explicit methods for aggregating participants' responses (see Box 1).

Box 1—Features of consensus methods	
Anonymity	To avoid dominance; achieved by use of a questionnaire in Delphi and private ranking in nominal groups
Iteration	Processes occur in "rounds", allowing individuals to change their opinions
Controlled feedback	Showing the distribution of the group's response (indicating to each individual their own previous response in Delphi)
Statistical group response	Expressing judgement using summary measures of the full group response, giving more information than a simple consensus statement

Adapted from Pill[6] and Rowe *et al.*[8]

The methods described

The Delphi process

The Delphi process takes its name from the Delphic oracles' skills of interpretation and foresight and has been used widely in health research within the fields of technology assessment, education and training, priority setting, developing nursing and clinical practice, workforce planning, forecasting and health service organisation.[1] The procedure enables a large group of experts to be contacted cheaply, usually by mail, using a self-administered questionnaire (though computer communications have also been used), with few geographical limitations on the sample. The process proceeds in a series of rounds as follows:

- Round 1: either relevant individuals are invited to provide opinions on a specific matter, based on their knowledge and experience, or the team undertaking the Delphi exercise expresses its opinions on a specific matter and selects suitable experts to participate in subsequent questionnaire rounds

  The opinions are then grouped together under a limited number of headings and statements, then drafted for circulation to all participants in the form of a questionnaire
- Round 2: participants rank their agreement with each statement in the questionnaire

  The rankings are subsequently summarised by the research team and included in a repeat version of the questionnaire
- Round 3: participants re-rank their agreement with each statement in the questionnaire, with the opportunity to change their scores in view of the group's response

  The re-rankings are summarised and assessed for the degree of consensus: if an acceptable degree of consensus is obtained, the process may cease with final results fed back to participants; if not, the third round is repeated.

In addition to scoring their agreement with statements, respondents are commonly asked to rate the confidence or certainty with which they express their opinions.

The nominal group technique

The nominal group technique uses a highly structured meeting to gather information from relevant experts (usually nine to 12 in number) about a given issue. The technique consists of two rounds in which panellists rate, discuss and then re-rate a series of items or questions. The method was developed in the United States in the 1960s and has been applied to problems in social services, education, government and industry.[1] In the context of health care the method has commonly been used to examine the appropriateness of clinical interventions, education and training, in practice development, for identifying measures for clinical trials and other research studies and to identify priorities in nursing, cancer care, primary care and health promotion.

A nominal group meeting is facilitated either by an expert on the topic[2] or a credible non-expert[3] and is structured as follows:

- Reviews of the relevant literature are provided to participants before the meeting

- Participants spend several minutes writing down their views about each topic in question
- Each participant, in turn, contributes one idea to the facilitator, who records it on a flip chart
- Similar suggestions are grouped together, where appropriate. There is a group discussion to clarify and evaluate each idea
- Each participant privately ranks each idea (round 1)
- The ranking is tabulated and presented
- The overall ranking is discussed and re-ranked (round 2)
- The final rankings are tabulated and the results fed back to the participants.

Alongside the consensus process, there may be a non-participant observer collecting qualitative data on the nominal group. This approach has some features in common with focus groups. However, the nominal group technique focuses on a single goal (for example, definition of criteria to assess the appropriateness of a surgical intervention) and is less concerned with eliciting a range of ideas or the qualitative analysis of the group process *per se* than is the case in focus groups.

Methodological issues

Who should participate?

There can be few hard and fast rules about who to include, except that each participant must be justifiable as in some way "expert" on the matter under discussion. Clearly, for studies concerned with defining criteria for a clinical intervention, the most appropriate experts will be clinicians practising in the field under consideration. Where the discussion concerns matters of general interest, such as health service priorities, participants should include non-clinical health professionals and should also allow for the expression of lay opinions.

Murphy et al.[4] devote a full chapter to the issue of participants in consensus methods, summarising the evidence on a number of important factors – group size, composition and personal and professional characteristics of participants. Their general finding is that there is insufficient evidence to provide clear guidance on many of these issues. However, they offer some guidance suggesting that personal characteristics should have relatively little influence provided the group is of sufficient size, that participants' status may affect group dynamics and that the formal methods should be designed to mitigate these effects. They also note that clinical specialty has an important influence in judgements of clinical appropriateness, and that study findings should be interpreted in the light of panel composition.

How should agreement be defined?

The term "agreement" can take two forms, which need to be distinguished: first, the extent to which each respondent *agrees with the issue* or statement under consideration (typically rated on a numerical or categorical scale), and second, the extent to which respondents *agree with each other* – the *consensus element* of these studies (typically assessed by statistical measures of dispersion).

It should be made clear to each participant that they need not conform to the group view – though, in the nominal group technique, those with atypical opinions (in comparison to the rest of the group) may face critical questioning of their views from other panel members. In a Delphi exercise, the researcher undertaking the study may ask participants that they have defined as outliers (for example, those in the lower and upper quartiles) to provide written justification for their responses.

How should agreement be measured?

Agreement with statements is usually summarised using the median and consensus is usually assessed using interquartile ranges for ordinal scales. In other contexts, for example, if a Delphi process is used to estimate probabilities of disease progression, the median of participants' responses may be taken as the group's estimate. The range or upper and lower quartiles may be used to express uncertainty around this estimate and may be adopted as extreme values during sensitivity analyses in decision analyses using these estimates. A more sophisticated measure of agreement used in some studies is the Kappa statistic.[5]

For nominal groups, rules have been developed to assess agreement when statements have been ranked on a 9-point scale. In an example where participants are rating appropriateness of interventions (where 0 = inappropriate and 9 = appropriate) the scale can be broken down so that scores 1–3 represent a region where participants feel that the intervention is not indicated; scores 4–6 represent a region where experts are equivocal; and scores 7–9 represent a region where participants feel intervention is indicated. The first rule is based on where the scores fall on the ranking scale: if all ratings fall within one of these pre-defined regions, there is said to be *strict* agreement. An alternative *relaxed* definition of agreement exists when all ratings fall within any 3-point region. This may be treated as agreement, in that all ratings are within an acceptable range, but the group opinion is ambiguous as to whether intervention is indicated or not.

The second rule tests whether extreme rankings are having an undue influence on the final results, and involves first, assessing the strict and relaxed definitions including all ratings for each statement and then assessing the strict and relaxed definitions excluding one extreme high and one extreme low rating for each statement.

How should the results of each round be fed back to participants?

Summary statistics may be fed back to participants at each round along with fuller indications of the distribution of responses to each statement in the form of tables of the proportions ranking at each point on the scale, histograms or other graphical representations of the range. Evidence suggests that it is more useful to feedback some information on the reasons for divergent views than simply to feed back ratings.

How should the accuracy of the answer obtained be assessed?

The existence of a consensus does not mean that the "correct" answer has been found – there is the danger of deriving collective ignorance rather than wisdom. The nominal group is not a replacement either for rigorous scientific reviews of published reports or for original research, but rather a means of identifying current medical opinion and areas of disagreement. For Delphi surveys, Pill recommends that the results should, where possible, be matched to observable events.[6]

Validity and applicability

Reviewing studies that compared group decision-making methods, Murphy *et al.* concluded that formal methods generally performed as well or better than informal methods.[4] However, it is difficult to tell which of the formal methods is best. Earlier reviews by Pill[6] and by Gerth and Smith[7] showed no clear evidence in favour of meeting-based methods over Delphi, although Rowe et al.[8] suggest that Delphi is generally inferior to the nominal group. This last conclusion is qualified by stating that the degree of inferiority is small, which is due more to practical than to theoretical difficulties.

There has been an active debate on the validity of the Delphi method. Sackman argued that the Delphi method fails to meet the standards normally set for scientific methods,[9] though his critique focused more on past poor quality studies rather than fundamental inadequacies of the method itself. He also argued that the method forces consensus and is weakened by not allowing participants to discuss issues. Murphy et al. offer some support for this position, suggesting that convergence of opinions during a Delphi exercise may have more to do with participants conforming to group norms than other influences, since the amount of information fed back tends to be limited.[4]

Applications of consensus methods

The earlier discussion of Delphi and NGT identified the contexts in which these approaches have been used in medical and health services research. They have been used predominantly in situations where there is conflicting or no evidence on which to base decisions or where the current evidence is of a form unsuitable for synthesis using conventional statistical methods. The Delphi approach may be most appropriately used where opinions are being sought – that is, where there is little or no role for evidence. Examples of these types of situation might be eliciting professional and public opinions on the principles for setting health priorities,[10] defining the clinical capabilities expected of health professionals, or projecting long-term care needs for particular client groups where there has been considerable uncertainty (for example, for cases of HIV and AIDS[11]). In contrast, the NGT would be most appropriate in situations where experts' opinions are being sought, but where there also exists a body of relevant evidence that participants should integrate into their decision-making processes. Thus each of the examples used for the Delphi approach could also use the NGT. However, the question posed might be slightly different – for example, rather than seeking opinion on principles for setting priorities, the question might be: "Which priorities should be adopted, taking into account evidence on effectiveness and cost of interventions?" Hence, opinion is being elicited, but current evidence is also incorporated. The nominal group technique seems particularly well adapted to the development of clinical guidelines, in that the approach uses the available evidence (evidence of all types rather than randomised controlled trials, as is the case for meta-analysis) but also allows for insight to be derived from the experience of relevant experts.

Murphy et al.[4] developed a conceptual model identifying five components of consensus development, grouped according to whether they were concerned with inputs, process or output (see Figure 1).

Three additional dimensions were identified. These were:

• planning, which included selection of the appropriate method (perhaps using the rule identified above, where Delphi might be used where only opinions are being sought and NGT where evidence is assessed as well as expert opinion) and consideration of the case for modification to the standard designs. At this stage, decisions over the number and type of participants to invite, the quantity and form of information to be provided, rules to be adopted for the interaction (including whether to hold a meeting,

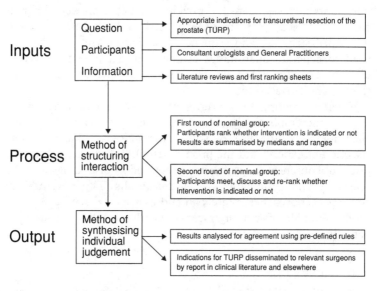

FIGURE 1—*Five components of consensus development (adapted from Jones and Hunter, 1995[12] and Murphy* et al., *1998[4])*

the number of meetings, the form the feedback should take and so on). Clearly, the majority of this activity will occur before participants are involved. However, they may have an input into how the results of each round should be fed back and how and where the output from the process should be presented;

- individual judgement, that is what participants do before meeting or before feedback of group opinion. In Delphi, this is Round 1. In NGT, this involves reading prepared materials such as literature reviews and, in some modifications of the NGT, the initial rating exercise;
- group interaction – in Delphi, this would include the effect of the group's response and in the NGT would involve meeting, discussion and possibly a change in participants' original judgements.

Conclusion

Consensus methods, in particular Delphi, have been described as methods of "last resort"[13] Even their advocates have warned against overselling them[14] and suggest that they should be regarded more as methods for structuring group communication on a question, than as a means for providing definitive answers. There is clearly a danger that since each method has evolved a well-developed structure and sequence of activities, and can often be used to generate quantitative estimates of agreement, they may lead the casual observer to place greater reliance on their results than might be warranted.

When presenting the findings of Delphi and nominal group studies, the emphasis should be on a clear justification for using such methods, the use of sound methodology (including the selection of experts and the precise definition of target acceptable levels of consensus), appropriate presentation of findings and the relevance and systematic use of the results. The output from consensus approaches is rarely an end in itself. Dissemination and implementation of such findings are the ultimate aim of consensus activities.

Further reading

Murphy MK, Black NA, Lamping DL, McKee CM, Sanderson CFB, Ashkam J, Marteau T. Consensus development methods, and their use in clinical guideline development. *Health Technology Assessment* 1998:2 (3).

References

1 Fink A, Kosecoff J, Chassin M, Brook RH. Consensus methods: characteristics and guidelines for use. *American Journal of Public Health* 1984;**74**:979–83.
2 Delbeq A, Van de Ven A. A group process model for problem identification and program planning. *Journal of Applied Behavioural Science* 1971;7:467–92.
3 Glaser EM. Using behavioural science strategies for defining the state-of-the-art. *Journal of Applied and Behavioural Sciences* 1980;**16**:79–92.
4 Murphy MK, Black NA, Lamping DL, McKee CM, Sanderson CFB, Ashkam J, Marteau T. Consensus development methods, and their use in clinical guideline development. *Health Technology Assessment* 1998;**2**(3).
5 Altman DC. *Practical statistics for medical research*. London: Chapman and Hall, 1991.
6 Pill J. The Delphi method: substance, context, a critique and an annotated bibliography. *Socio-Economic Planning Science* 1971;**5**:57–71.
7 Gerth W, Smith ME. The Delphi technique. Background for use in probability estimation. *Human Health Economics* MHHD. Merck and Co., September 1991.
8 Rowe G, Wright G, Bolger F. Delphi: a re-evaluation of research and theory. *Technological Forecasting and Social Change* 1991;**39**:235–51.
9 Sackman H. *Delphi Critique*. Lexington, MA: Lexington Books, 1975.
10 Moscovice I, Armstrong P, Shortell S. Health services research for decision-makers: the use of the Delphi technique to determine health priorities. *Journal of Health Politics, Policy and Law* 1988;**2**:388–410.
11 Chin J, Sato PA, Mann JM. Projections of HIV infections and AIDS cases to the year 2000. *Bulletin of the World Health Organisation* 1990;**68**:1–11.
12 Jones JMG, Hunter D. Consensus methods for medical and health services research. *Br Med J* 1995;**311**:376–80.
13 Coates JF. In defense of Delphi: a review of Delphi assessment, expert opinion, forecasting and group process by H. Sackman. *Technological Forecasting and Social Change* 1975:7:193–4.
14 Linstone HA. The Delphi technique In: Fowles RB. ed. *Handbook of Futures Research*. Westport, CT : Greenwood Press, 1978.

6 Using case studies in health services and policy research

JUSTIN KEEN, TIM PACKWOOD

Introduction

The medical approach to understanding disease has traditionally drawn heavily on qualitative data and, in particular, on case studies to illustrate important or interesting phenomena. Much of the everyday work of doctors and other health professionals still involves decisions that are qualitative rather than quantitative in nature; a tradition maintained by regular case study reports in the *BMJ* and other leading medical journals. This chapter discusses the use of qualitative research methods, not in individual clinical care, but in case studies of wider health service changes. It is useful to understand the principles guiding the design and conduct of these studies, because they are used both by researchers and inspecting agencies, such as the Audit Commission in England and Wales and the General Accounting Office in the USA, to investigate the work of doctors and other health professionals. These studies might be expected, in time, to inform the methodological approach of the NHS's new Commission for Health Improvement.[1]

The next section will briefly outline the circumstances where case study research can usefully be undertaken in health service settings. Then, the ways in which qualitative methods are used within case studies are discussed. Illustrative examples are used to show how qualitative methods are applied.

Case study research

Doctors often find themselves asking important practical questions: should we be involved in the management of NHS Primary Care Groups? How can we cope with changes in practice in our local setting? There are, broadly, two ways in which such questions can usefully be addressed. One is to analyse the proposed policies themselves, by investigating whether they are internally consistent, and by using theoretical frameworks derived from previous research to predict their effects on the ground. The policies announced in *The New NHS*[1] and the current community care arrangements have been analysed in this way using economic and political science-based explanations of their likely consequences.[2,3]

The other approach, and the focus of this article, is to study implementation empirically. Empirical evaluative studies are concerned with placing a value on an intervention or policy change, and typically involve forming judgements about the appropriateness of the intervention for those concerned (and often by implication also for the health system as a whole), and whether the outputs and outcomes of the intervention are justified by their inputs and processes. Asking participants about their experiences, or observing them in meetings and other work settings, can provide rich data for descriptive and explanatory accounts of organisational processes, work practices, and the impact of change.

When is it appropriate to use case studies? Case studies are valuable where policy change is occurring in messy real world settings, and it is important to understand why such interventions succeed or fail. The key problem is that the ways in which policies are formulated and promulgated means that researchers have no control over events. As a result, experimental designs are typically not feasible, and even the opportunities for rigorous comparison using observational designs can be limited. Worse, an intervention may be ill-defined, at least at the outset – think of the uncertainty about the nature of Primary Care Groups in the English NHS before they were introduced, or of the complex organisational changes taking place in US care – and so cannot easily be distinguished from the general environment. Even where it is well defined, an intervention may not have costs and effects that are easily captured. For example, the networking and other elements of the NHS information technology strategy are well defined, but might be expected to exert their effects over different timescales, in many different places and on different groups of people.

Another reason to consider case studies is that questions about policy and practice touch on local and national health politics. Many interventions will typically depend for their success on the involvement of several different interested parties, so it is often necessary to be sensitive to issues of collaboration and conflict. Each party may have a legitimate, but different, interpretation of events. Capturing these different views is often best achieved using interviews or other qualitative methods within a case study design. And, for political and other reasons, it is often not clear at the outset whether an intervention will be fully implemented by the end of a study period. One has only to think of accounts of the problems faced in implementing computer systems in health care[4] – yet study of these failures may provide invaluable clues that help to shape future policies. In short, the strength of good case study designs is that they can cope with, and provide insights into, complex real world developments, with the "case" providing a source of explanations for wider developments.

Design of case studies

As noted earlier, case studies employing qualitative methods are used by bodies that regulate public services. Examples include the work of the National Audit Office (NAO)[5] and the Audit Commission[6] in the UK, and audit offices and regulatory bodies in other countries.[7,8] Case studies have also been used in evaluations, including studies of the introduction of general management[9] and business process re-engineering[10] in hospitals, and of general practice fundholding[11,12] in the UK, and of total quality initiatives in the USA.[13] All used one or more qualitative methods including interviews, analysis of documentation and non-participant obser-vation of meetings.

These studies have a number of common features. Each one involved identifying research questions that stemmed from con-cerns about the implications of new policies, or from concerns about implementation "on the ground", or from claims about new management theories such as re-engineering. Case studies may well be prospective, examining the implementation of policies over a period of time. This was the case with resource management, business process re-engineering and total purchasing, all of which are discussed below.

Once a broad research question has been identified, there are two approaches to the design of case study research, either of which may be appropriate depending on the circumstances. In the first, precise questions are posed at the outset of the research and data collection and analysis are directed towards answering them. These studies are typically constructed to allow comparisons to be drawn.[14] The comparison may be between different approaches to implementation, or between sites where an intervention is taking place and ones where normal practice prevails. In a recent study of clinical audit in the therapy professions,[15] themes regarding the development and practice of audit were identified from interviews with key informants and then used in constructing interview schedules to enable comparison between the case study and other sites.

Another example is provided by the study of total purchasing pilot general practices by Mays *et al.*[16] This study of an extension of the general practitioner fundholding model could not be experimental in terms of matched comparisons with non-pilots, or hope to apply other controls preventing contamination by external factors. But comparisons could be made within the sample, for example between different sizes of practice or different waves of pilots. It was also possible to focus on particular topics (risk management, financial management) or services (mental health, maternity) and thereby highlight the emerging lessons for future NHS policy for primary care.

The second approach is more open, and in effect starts by asking very broad questions: "What is happening here, what are the important features and relationships that will affect the outcome of this policy?" This approach can form the early stages of the more focused approach discussed above. The early fieldwork, often using interviews and observation of meetings, is designed to generate data that are then used to identify and refine specific research questions inductively. This type of design, in which detailed research questions emerge during the course of the study, has been advocated for general use in the study of the impact of government policies in the health system.[17] In some ways, it is similar to the way in which clinical consultations are conducted, in that it involves initial exploration followed by progress over time towards a diagnosis inferred from the available data. An example of this approach was the evaluation of resource management (RM) in NHS hospitals,[18] which investigated the progress of six pilot hospitals in implementing new management arrangements, focusing particularly on identifying ways in which doctors and general managers could jointly control the allocation and commitment of resources.

At the outset, the nature of RM was unclear. A similar problem faced the researchers evaluating total purchasing. Sites were charged with finding ways of involving doctors in management, but how this would be achieved and, if achieved, how successful it would be in improving patient care, were open questions. The researchers selected major specialties within each site, and conducted interviews with relevant staff, observed meetings and analysed documentation (see Box 1). Over time, the data were used to develop a framework that captured the essential features of RM, and the framework was then used to evaluate each site's progress with implementation (see Box 2). A more recent example of this approach is provided by a study of the impact of business process re-engineering (BPR) in a teaching hospital.[10] The study had to

Box 1—Evaluation of the resource management initiative[18]

- Six hospitals, a mix of teaching and non-teaching
- Focus on major specialties: general surgery and general medicine
- Mix of qualitative and quantitative methods
- Methods and data sources independent of each other
- Qualitative methods included interviews, non-participant observation of meetings and analysis of documents

Box 2—Analytical framework: five inter-related elements of resource management[18]

- Commitment to resource management by the relevant personnel at each level in the organisation
- Devolution of authority for the management of resources
- Collaboration within and between disciplines in securing the objectives of resource management
- Management infrastructure, particularly in terms of organisation structure and provision of information
- A clear focus for the resource management strategy

follow and adapt to the dynamics of the BPR programme, as it changed over the period of the case study in response to experience and external influences.

The process of selecting sites for study is central to the case study approach. Researchers have developed a number of selection strategies, the objectives of which, as in any good research study, are to ensure that misinterpretation of results is avoided as far as possible. Because resources for case study work are usually limited, it is necessary to design a "purposive" sample that is typical of the phenomenon being investigated, where a specific theory can be tested, or where cases will confirm or refute a hypothesis.[19] Researchers can benefit from expert advice from those with knowledge of the subject being investigated, and can usefully build the possibility of testing findings at further sites into the initial research design. Replication of results across sites helps to ensure that findings are not due to idiosyncratic features of particular sites.

The next step is to select data collection methods, ensuring that the process is driven by criteria of validity and reliability.[20] A distinctive, though not unique, feature of case study research is the use of multiple methods and sources of evidence to establish construct validity.[21] The total purchasing study provides an example (see Box 3). The use of particular methods is discussed in other chapters of the book. Here it is noted that case studies often use "triangulation"[22] (see Chapter 9) to maximise confidence in the validity of findings. In triangulation, all data items are corroborated from at least one other source and normally also via another method of data collection. Any one method can, arguably, produce results of weaker validity than a combination. Using different methods and sources helps to address this problem, and can

---

Box 3—Methods used in the national evaluation of total purchasing pilots[16]

- Face-to-face interviews with key players
- Diary cards to samples of key players
- Postal questionnaires
- Telephone interviews
- Documentary analysis
- Quantitative data analysis (including NHS routine data)

strengthen researchers' beliefs in the validity of their observations. This said, reservations have been expressed about the use of triangulation in qualitative research,[21] given that different methods and sources of data will tend to provide different sorts of insights rather than contribute to a single, accumulating picture. Some studies have, by contrast, used comparison of case study data with that from a larger sample to explore how far findings might be strengthened and generalised. The evaluation of total purchasing[16] employed this strategy, using survey as well as case study site data. The key point here is that the case study approach, properly used, can be viewed as a strategy for combining data and methods systematically in order to validate findings.

Another example of the central concern of case studies with establishing validity is provided in a study of purchaser–provider contracting for community health services.[23] The purpose of the study was to gather information about the processes involved in contracting in the NHS internal market. A small number of sites were chosen, the selection of sites being based in part on different organisational structures and approaches to purchasing to allow for broad comparison of experiences. Observations of meetings were recorded, verbatim notes were made of discussions in situ, and documents were obtained about all stages of the contracting process. Interviews were held with patients and users of health services, and an interview survey of GPs was conducted. The data obtained using each method were analysed separately and then compared with one another across different methods and study sites.

Whatever the details, the collection of data should be directed towards the development of an analytical framework that will facilitate interpretation of findings. Again, there are several ways in which this might be done. Sometimes data are collected in order to test specific hypotheses. In the evaluation of resource management, in contrast, there was no obvious pre-existing theory that could be applied: the development of a framework during the study was crucial to help organise data and evaluate findings. The framework was not imposed on the data, but derived from it in an iterative process over the course of the evaluation; each was used to refine the other over time. Possibilities for testing emerging findings can be built into case study design – for example, by feedback in report or workshop form to participants or knowledgeable informants, or by using further small-scale case studies.

The investigator is finally left with the difficult task of making a judgement about the findings of a study and determining its wider implications. The purpose of the steps followed in designing and building the case study is to maximise confidence in the findings, but interpretation inevitably involves value judgements and the danger of bias. The extent to which research findings can be assembled into a single coherent account of events varies; individual cases may exhibit common characteristics or fare very differently. In some circumstances widely differing opinions of participants are themselves very important, and should be reflected in any report. The case study approach enables the researcher to gauge confidence in both the internal and external validity of the findings, and make comments with the appropriate assurance or with reservations.

Conclusion

The complexity of the issues that health professionals have to address and increasing recognition by policy makers, academics and practitioners of the value of case studies in evaluating health service interventions, suggest that the use of such studies is likely to increase in the future. Their most important use may be by regulators, possibly including bodies in the NHS such as the Commission for Health Improvement,[1] so they will become part of the machinery whereby doctors and other clinicians are held to account for their work. In policy research, qualitative methods can be used within case study design to address many practical and policy questions that impinge on the lives of clinicians, particularly where those questions are concerned with how or why events or initiatives take a particular course.

Further reading

Yin R. *Case study research: design and methods.* Second edition. Newbury Park, CA: Sage, 1994.

References

1 Secretary of State for Health. *The new NHS: modern, dependable.* Cm 3807. London: Stationery Office, 1997.
2 Klein R. ed. *Implementing the White Paper: pitfalls and opportunities.* London: King's Fund, 1998.
3 Wistow G, Knapp M, Hardy B *et al. Social care markets: progress and prospects.* Buckingham: Open University Press, 1996.

4 National Audit Office. *NHS executive: the purchase of the Read codes and the management of the Centre for Coding and Classification.* HC 607, Session 1997–98. London: Stationery Office, 1998.

5 National Audit Office. *Cost over-runs, funding problems and delays on Guy's Hospital phase III development.* HC 761, Session 1997–98. London: Stationery Office, 1998.

6 Audit Commission. *Higher purchase: commissioning specialised services in the NHS.* London: Stationery Office, 1997.

7 Gray A. *Budgeting, auditing and evaluation: functions and integration in seven governments.* New Brunswick, NJ: Transaction, 1993.

8 Pollitt C, Girre X, Lonsdale J, Mul R, Summa H, Waerness M. *Performance or compliance? Performance audit and public management in five countries.* Oxford: Oxford University Press, 1999.

9 Pollitt C, Harrison S, Hunter D, Marnoch G. The reluctant managers: clinicians and budgets in the NHS. *Financial Accountability and Management* 1988;4:213–33.

10 Packwood T, Pollitt C, Roberts S. Good medicine: a case study of business process re-engineering in a hospital. *Policy and Politics,* 1998;26:401–15.

11 Laughlin R. Empirical research in accounting: alternative approaches and a case for 'middle range' thinking. *Accounting, Auditing and Accountability Journal* 1997:10; 622–48.

12 Laughlin R, Broadbent J, Willig-Atherton H. Recent financial and administrative changes in GP practices: initial experiences and effects. *Accounting, Auditing and Accountability Journal* 1994;7:96–124.

13 Berwick D, Roessner A, Godfrey J. *Curing health care.* San Francisco, CA: Jossey Bass:191.

14 St Leger A, Schneider H, Walsworth-Bell J. *Evaluating health services effectiveness.* Milton Keynes: Open University Press, 1992.

15 Kogan M, Redfern S. *Making use of clinical audit.* Buckingham: Open University Press, 1995.

16 Mays N, Goodwin N, Killoran A, Malbon G. *Total purchasing: a step towards primary care groups.* London: King's Fund, 1998.

17 Pollitt C, Harrison S, Hunter D, Marnoch G. No hiding place: on the discomforts of researching the contemporary policy process. *Journal of Social Policy* 1990;19:169–90.

18 Packwood T, Keen J, Buxton M. *Hospitals in transition: the resource management experiment.* Milton Keynes: Open University Press, 1991.

19 Patton M. *Qualitative evaluation and research methods.* Second edition. Newbury Park, CA: Sage, 1990.

20 Yin R. *Case study research: design and methods.* Second edition. Newbury Park, CA: Sage, 1994.

21 Silverman D. *Interpreting qualitative research.* London: Sage, 1993.

22 Jick T. Mixing qualitative and quantitative methods: triangulation in action. *Administrative Sciences Quarterly* 1979;24:602–11.

23 Flynn R, Williams G, Pickard S. *Markets and networks: contracting in community health services.* Buckingham: Open University Press, 1996.

7 Using qualitative methods in health-related action research

JULIENNE MEYER

The barriers to the uptake of the findings of traditional quantitative biomedical research in clinical practice are increasingly being recognised.[1,2] Certain forms of qualitative research may make it easier for research to influence day-to-day practice. The style of research known as action research is particularly suited to identifying problems in clinical practice and helping to develop potential solutions in order to improve practice.[3] For this reason, action research is increasingly being employed in health-related settings. Although not synonymous with qualitative research, action research usually draws on the types of qualitative methods described in Chapters 2, 3 and 4 of this book. Action research projects are frequently written up as case studies, but this approach to research is distinct from the types of case study discussed in Chapter 6.

What is action research?

Like qualitative research in general, action research is not easily defined. It is a style of research rather than a specific method. First used in 1946 by Kurt Lewin, a social scientist concerned with inter-group relations and minority problems in the USA, it is now identified with research in which the researchers work explicitly *with* and *for* people rather than undertake research *on* them.[4] Action research appears to be gaining credibility in a variety of practice-based disciplines, particularly within the health care professions. Its strength lies in its focus on generating solutions to practical

59

problems and its ability to empower practitioners – getting them to engage with research and subsequent "development" or implementation activities. Practitioners can be involved when they choose to research their own practice[5] or when an outside researcher is engaged to help them to identify problems, seek and implement potential solutions, and systematically monitor and reflect on the process and outcomes of change.[6,7]

The term "action research" tends to be used loosely. However, most definitions incorporate three important elements, namely its participatory character, its democratic impulse, and its simultaneous contribution both to social science and social change.[8]

Participation in action research

Participation is fundamental to action research; it is an approach which demands that participants perceive the need to change and are willing to play an active role both in the research and change process. Whilst all research requires willing subjects, the level of commitment required of those involved in an action research study goes beyond simply agreeing to answer questions or to be observed. The clear-cut demarcation between "researcher" and "researched" found in other types of research may not be apparent in action research. The research design or strategy is *negotiated* with participants in a continuous process in an action research study, making obtaining informed consent at the outset problematic. Action researchers, therefore, need to agree an ethical code of practice with the participants.[9] Participation in the research and in the process of change can be threatening, and conflicts may arise in the course of the research, as a number of studies have shown.[10, 11] For example, in one action research study[6] the process of asking for suggestions for improvements and honestly feeding them back to participants had a profound effect on the dynamics of a multidisciplinary team. Not all participants in the study felt comfortable questioning their own practice and examining their own roles and responsibilities. Indeed, the nurse in charge found it particularly threatening and this resulted in her seeking employment elsewhere.[9] Where an outside researcher is working with practitioners it is important to obtain their trust and agree rules on the control of data and their use, and on how potential conflict will be resolved within the project. The way in which such rules are agreed demonstrates a second important feature of action research, namely its democratic impulse.

Democracy in action research

Action research is concerned with intervening to change and improve practice whether in health, education or any other area of life.[12] It engages participants in the struggle for more rational, just, democratic and fulfilling forms of "service". As such, it can be seen as a form of "critical" social science.[13] This philosophical under-pinning is a key difference between action research and more traditional case study approaches. "Democracy" in action research usually requires participants to be seen as equals of the researcher. The researcher works as a facilitator of change, consulting with participants not only on the action process, but also on how it will be evaluated. One benefit of designing a study in conjunction with practitioners is that it can make the research process and outcomes more meaningful to practitioners, by rooting them in the reality of day-to-day practice.

Throughout the study, findings are fed back to participants for validation and to inform decisions about the next stage of the study. This formative style of research is thus responsive to events as they naturally occur in the field and frequently entails collaborative spirals of planning, acting, observing, reflecting and re-planning (see Figure 1).[14] These action–reflection spirals are characteristic of any action research study. McNiff[14] visually depicts action research as a three dimensional tree of spirals, allowing for smaller "spin-off spirals" to branch out from larger spirals of activity. This

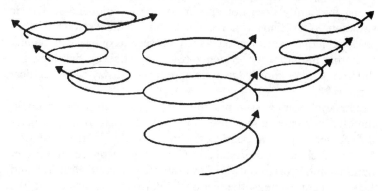

FIGURE 1—*Action–reflection spirals*

illustrates how practitioners engaging in action research can address many different problems at one time without losing sight of the main issue. It also captures the frequently seemingly chaotic nature of change in organisations and practice settings.

However, as has already been noted, the open feedback of findings to participants can be, and often is, very threatening. Democratic practice is not always a feature of health care settings. Care needs to be taken in undertaking democratic action research in such settings. An action researcher needs to be able to work across traditional boundaries (for example, between professionals, health and social care, and between hospital and community care) and juggle different, sometimes competing agendas. Excellent interpersonal skills, in addition to research ability, are clearly of paramount importance in action research.

Contribution to both social science and social change

The focus on practice and on change, and the greater level of involvement by participants in the research process, opens action research to the challenge of being "unscientific". This is compounded by the fact that action research in health care settings has tended to utilise a range of qualitative methods rather than the quantitative methods associated with clinical, biological and epidemiological research. Yet, there is increasing concern about the theory–practice gap in clinical practice in which practitioners have to rely on their intuition and experience since traditional scientific knowledge, for example, the results of randomised controlled trials, frequently does not appear to fit the uniqueness of their situation. (Clinicians will recognise this as the exercise of professional judgement.) Action research is seen as one way of dealing with this limitation of evidence-based practice by developing a different kind of knowledge more appropriate to day-to-day clinical settings.[4, 8]

The level of interest in practitioner-led research is increasing in the UK, in part as a response to recent proposals to "modernise" the National Health Service through the development of new forms of clinical governance.[15] Clinical governance and other national initiatives in the UK (for example, the NHS Research and Development Strategy, the National Centre for Clinical Audit, the NHS Centre for Reviews and Dissemination, the Cochrane

Collaboration, and Centres for Evidence Based Practice) emphasise that research and development should be the business of every clinician. It is argued[16] that practitioner-led research approaches, such as single case experimental designs,[17] reflective case studies[18] and reflexive action research,[19] are ideal research methods for clinicians concerned with improving the quality of patient care. In addition, these approaches are likely to generate findings that are more meaningful and useful to practitioners, thus reducing the theory–practice gap.

In considering the contribution of action research to knowledge, it is important to note that generalisations made from action research studies differ from those made on the basis of more conventional forms of research. To some extent, reports of action research studies rely on the reader to underwrite the account of the research by drawing on their own knowledge of human situations. It is, therefore, important, when reporting action research, to describe the work in its rich contextual detail. The researcher strives to include the participants' perspective on the data by feeding back findings to participants and incorporating their responses as new data in the final report. In addition, the onus is on the researcher to make his/her own values and beliefs explicit in the account of the research so that any biases are evident. This can be facilitated by writing self-reflective field notes when undertaking the research. According to Carr and Kemmis,[8] a successful report can be characterised by "the shock of recognition" – the quality of the account enables readers to assess its relevance to themselves and their own practice situations. The systematic feeding back of findings throughout an action research study, makes it possible to check the accuracy of the account with participants. However, interpreting the relevance of the findings to any other practice situation ultimately rests with the reader (see Chapter 9 for more on issues of validity and relevance in qualitative research).

The strength of action research lies in its ability to influence practice positively in the course of the study, whilst, at the same time, systematically gathering data to share with a wider audience. The involvement of practitioners in this process ensures not only more likelihood of discovering successful solutions to everyday problems, but also of obtaining a different type of data that is, arguably, more relevant and meaningful to practitioners.

However, change is problematic and, whilst action research lends itself well to the discovery of solutions, its success should not be judged solely in terms of the size of change achieved or the immediate implementation of solutions. Instead, success can often be viewed in relation to what has been learnt from the experience of undertaking the work. For instance, a study that set out to explore the care of older people in A and E departments[20] did not result in much change in the course of the study. However, the lessons learnt from the research were reviewed in the context of national policy and research and carefully fed back to those working in the organisation and, as a result, changes have already been made within the organisation to act on the study's recommendations. For instance, some positive changes were achieved in the course of the study (for example, the introduction of specialist discharge posts in A and E), but the study also shed light on continuing gaps in care and issues that needed to be improved in future developments. Participants identified that the role of the action researcher had enabled greater understanding and communication between two services (the A and E Department and the Department of Medicine for Elderly People), and that this had left both better equipped for future joint working. In other words, the solutions emerged from the process of undertaking the research.

Different types of action research

Under the same broad heading, there are many different types of action research. Hart and Bond[3] suggest that there are some key characteristics, which not only distinguish action research from other methodologies, but which also determine the range of approaches to action research. They present a typology of action research identifying four basic types: experimental, organisational, professionalising and empowering (see Box 1). They suggest that each type embodies a different theoretical perspective on society.

Whilst this typology is useful in understanding the wide range of action research, its multi-dimensional nature means that it is not particularly easy to classify individual studies. For instance, whilst a study might be classified as "empowering" because of its "bottom-up approach" in relation to the fourth distinguishing criteria of "change intervention" (see Box 2), the other distinguishing criteria may be used to classify the same study as a different action research type (experimental, organisational or professionalising). This situation is most likely to occur if the researcher and

Box 1—Action research typology (reproduced with permission from Hart and Bond, 1995)[3]

Action research type: Distinguishing criteria	Consensus model of society / Rational social management / Experimental	Organisational	Professionalising	Conflict model of society / Structural change / Empowering
1 Educative base	Re-education	Re-education/training	Reflective practice	Consciousness-raising
	Enhancing social science/administrative control and social change towards consensus	Enhancing managerial control and organisational change towards consensus	Enhancing professional control and individual's ability to control work situation	Enhancing user-control and shifting balance of power; structural change towards pluralism
	Inferring relationship between behaviour and output; identifying causal factors in group dynamics	Overcoming resistance to change/restructuring balance of power between managers and workers	Empowering professional groups; advocacy on behalf of patients/clients	Empowering oppressed groups
2 Individuals in groups	Social scientific bias/researcher focused	Managerial bias/client focused	Practitioner focused	User/practitioner focused
	Closed group, controlled, selection made by researcher for purposes of measurement/ inferring relationship between cause and effect	Work groups and/or mixed groups of managers and workers	Professional(s) and/or (interdisciplinary) professional group/negotiated team boundaries	Fluid groupings, self selecting or natural boundary or open/closed by negotiation
	Fixed membership	Selected membership	Shifting membership	Fluid membership

Box 1—Continued

Action research type: Distinguishing criteria	Consensus model of society / Rational social management / Experimental	Organisational	Professionalising	Conflict model of society / Structural change / Empowering
3 Problem focus	Problem emerges from the interaction of social science theory and social problems Problem relevant for social science/management interests Success defined in terms of social sciences	Problem defined by most powerful group; some negotiation with workers Problem relevant for management/social science interests Success defined by sponsors	Problem defined by professional group; some negotiation with users Problem emerges from professional practice/experience Contested, professionally determined definitions of success	Emerging and negotiated definition of problem by less powerful group(s) Problem emerges from members' practice/experience Competing definitions of success accepted and expected
4 Change intervention	Social science, experimental intervention to test theory and/or generate theory Problem to be solved in terms of research aims	Top-down, directed change towards predetermined aims Problem to be solved in terms of management aims	Professionally led, predefined, process-led Problem to be resolved in the interests of research-based practice and professionalisation	Bottom-up, underdetermined, process-led Problem to be explored as part of process of change, developing an understanding of meaning of issues in terms of problem and solution

Box 1—Continued

Action research type: Distinguishing criteria	Consensus model of society / Rational social management / Experimental	Organisational	→ Professionalising	→ Conflict model of society / Structural change / Empowering
5 Improvement and involvement	Towards controlled outcome and consensual definition of improvement	Towards tangible outcome and consensual definition of improvement	Towards improvement in practice defined by professionals and on behalf of users	Towards negotiated outcomes and pluralist definitions of improvement; account taken of vested interests
6 Cyclic processes	Research components dominant	Action and research components in tension; action dominated	Research and action components in tension; research dominated	Action components dominant
	Identifies causal processes that can be generalised	Identifies causal processes that are specific to problem context and/or can be generalised	Identifies causal processes that are specific to problem and/or can be generalised	Changes course of events; recognition of multiple influences upon change
	Time limited, task focused	Discrete cycle, rationalist, sequential	Spiral of cycles, opportunistic, dynamic	Open-ended, process driven
7 Research relationship, degree of collaboration	Experimenter/respondents	Consultant/researcher, respondent/participants	Practitioner or researcher/collaborators	Practitioner researcher/co-researchers/co-change agents
	Outside researcher as expert/research funding	Client pays an outside consultant — "they who pay the piper call the tune"	Outside resources and/or internally generated	Outside resources and/or internally generated
	Differentiated roles	Differentiated roles	Merged roles	Shared roles

practitioners hold differing views on the nature of society. This makes classification of single studies into any one type of action research problematic. Instead, it may be more fruitful to use this typology as a framework for critiquing individual studies and, in particular for thinking about how concepts are operationalised, the features of particular settings, and the contribution of the people within those settings to solutions.[21] It is worth noting that, over time, health-related action research appears to have moved away from "experimental" to more "empowering" models of research.[9] However, empowering models have to be used with care.[22] Health service organisations are frequently hierarchical rather than demo-cratic. As a result, changes based on notions of practitioner empowerment can frequently be frustrated. Somekh[23] reiterates this point, arguing that different occupational cultures can affect action research methodology. For this reason, she suggests that action research should be grounded in the values and discourse of the individual or group rather than rigidly adhering to a particular methodological perspective.

Action research in health care

At a time when there is increasing concern that research evidence is not sufficiently influencing practice development,[24] it is not surprising that action research is gaining credibility in health care settings.[25] For example, the Royal College of Physicians in England has become involved in an action research study, commissioned by the NHS Executive, which seeks to improve the practice of clinical audit. A central focus of this study is to explore the roles of clinicians, clinical audit staff and managers in implementing clinical audit and in determining how organisational problems can be overcome.[26] The interest in action research within health care settings can also be demonstrated by the recent commissioning of a methodological systematic review of the action research lit-erature, as part of the NHS Research and Development Programme. The intention behind this review is to provide guidance for funding agencies, policy makers and researchers on the criteria to use to judge the appropriateness of action research proposals and reports.

Since action research seeks to develop a process of change in practice contexts and emphasises the role of the practitioner as researcher, it allows research to become part of the clinician's everyday work. In many ways, its use is ideally suited to health services research and its popularity is likely to be sustained.

Ong[27] advocates the value of action research within health care settings on the basis of recent changes in the requirements of health care management and policy. She highlights the need for new, systematic approaches to encouraging user participation in health services. She suggests that "Rapid Appraisal" is an ideal method for engaging users in the development of health care policy and practice.[28] Rapid Appraisal is a type of action research, hitherto predominantly used in developing countries, which focuses on participatory methods to foster change, using ideas derived from the field of community development. Her book gives excellent detail not only on the philosophical and theoretical underpinnings of Rapid Appraisal, but also on how such a study might be conducted.[28]

Action research has also been used in hospital rather than wider community settings to facilitate closer partnerships between staff and users. In a study that focused on the introduction of lay participation in care within a general medical ward of a London teaching hospital, the action researcher worked for one year in a multi-disciplinary team (see Box 2).[6] In the course of the study, it emerged that in order to foster closer partnerships with users and carers, professionals needed to change their practice to work more collaboratively with one another. As a result, three main action–reflection spirals emerged in the project: reorganising the work of the ward, multi-disciplinary communication, and lay participation in care. Each action–reflection spiral generated related activities, otherwise known as spin-off spirals. For instance, stemming from the main lay participation in care action–reflection spiral, a spin-off spiral focused on the medical staff teaching patients more about their treatments.

A range of research methods was used, including depth interviews (see Chapter 2), questionnaires, documentary analysis and participant observation (see Chapter 4). Throughout the study, preliminary findings were fed back to participants through weekly team meetings to help guide the project. Whilst positive change was demonstrated over time, the analysis generated two main data sets on the health professionals' perceptions of lay participation in care and the difficulties encountered in changing practice.[29,30]

The value of using qualitative methods and an action research approach can best be demonstrated in relation to the data on the health professionals' perceptions of lay participation in care. Qualitative methods were used alongside quantitative methods such as attitudinal scales and self-administered questionnaires as part of a process of triangulation (see Chapter 9). As suggested in Chapter 1, qualitative methods can be useful in reinterpreting the findings from more quantitative methods. In this study, health professionals expressed extremely positive views about user and carer involvement when completing an attitude scale.[31] However, examination of their attitudes in interviews suggested that they had some serious doubts and concerns. Subsequent observation of

---

Box 2—Lay participation in care in a hospital setting: an action research study

Participation	Careful negotiation to recruit willing volunteers to examine practice and initiate lay participation in care "Bottom-up" approach to change via weekly team meetings Researcher as facilitator and multi-disciplinary team member
Democracy	Goal of empowering practitioners and lay people in this setting Working collaboratively with multi-disciplinary team Participants given "ownership" of the data to determine how it might be shared with wider audience
Contribution to social science and social change	Findings constantly fed back to practitioners, leading to changes (such as, improvements in inter-professional working) Dissemination of findings of local and national relevance
Evaluation methods	Case study of multi-disciplinary team on one general medical ward in London teaching hospital using: • qualitative methods to highlight key themes emerging in the project • quantitative methods for comparison of sub groups

---

Box 2—Continued

Main action–reflection spirals	Reorganising the work of the ward • Changes in patient care planning • New reporting system, including bed-side handover with patient • Introduction of modified form of primary nursing system Multi-disciplinary communication • Weekly team meetings instituted • Introduction of a handout for new staff and team communication sheet • Closer liaison with community nurses before discharge Lay participation in care • Development of resources for patient health education • Introduction of medicine reminder card system • Patient information leaflet inviting patients to participate in care
Results	Insights into health professionals' perceptions of lay participation in care Some positive changes achieved (e.g. improved attitudes to lay participation in care, patient education, improved ward organisation) Identified barriers to changing health care practice

their practice revealed that these doubts and concerns were inhibiting the implementation of lay participation. Previous research on health professionals' attitudes towards user and carer involvement had tended to rely solely on structured instruments and had found that health professionals hold generally positive attitudes towards it.[31-34] By contrast, using mixed methods, it was possible to explore the relationship between attitudes and practices and to explain what happened when lay participation was introduced into a practice setting. Findings suggested that, whilst current policy documents advocate lay participation in care, some health professionals were merely paying lip service to the concept and were also inadequately prepared to deliver it in practice. In addition, findings indicated that health professionals needed to learn to collaborate more closely with each other, by developing a common understanding and approach to patient care, in order to offer closer partnerships with users and carers.

Whilst one cannot generalise from a single case study, this research led to serious questioning of the value of previous quantitative research, which had suggested that health professionals hold positive attitudes towards lay participation in care. By using action research and working closely with practitioners to explore issues in a practical context, more insight was gained into how the rhetoric of policy might be better translated into reality.

Conclusion

Action research does not focus exclusively on user and carer involvement, though clearly its participatory principles make it an obvious choice to explore these issues. It can be used more widely, for example, to foster better practice across inter-professional boundaries and between different health care settings.[20,35] Action research can also be used by clinicians to research their own practice.[16] It is an eclectic approach to research, which draws on a variety of data collection methods. However, its focus on the process as well as the outcomes of change helps to explain the frequent use of qualitative methods by action researchers.

Further reading

Hart E, Bond M. *Action research for health and social care. A guide to practice.* Buckingham: Open University Press, 1995.
Susman GI, Evered RD. An assessment of the scientific merits of action research. *Administrative Science Quarterly* 1978;**23**:582–603.

References

1 Sackett DL, Richardson WS, Rosenberg W, Haynes RB. *Evidence-based medicine: how to practise and teach EBM.* Edinburgh: Churchill Livingstone, 1997.
2 Hicks C, Hennessy D. Mixed messages in nursing research: their contribution to the persisting hiatus between evidence and practice. *Journal of Advanced Nursing* 1997;**25**:595–601.
3 Hart E, Bond M. *Action research for health and social care: a guide to practice.* Buckingham: Open University Press, 1995.
4 Reason P, Rowan J. *Human inquiry: a sourcebook of new paradigm research.* Chichester: John Wiley and Sons, 1981.
5 Childs V, Franklin F and Kemp P. *Action research in social services and health care settings.* Cambridge: Anglia Polytechnic University, 1997.
6 Meyer JE. *Lay participation in care in a hospital setting: an action research study.* London: University of London, unpublished PhD thesis, 1995.

7 Titchen, A. *Changing nursing practice through action research.* Oxford: National Institute for Nursing, 1993.

8 Carr W, Kemmis S. *Becoming critical: education, knowledge and action research.* London: Falmer Press, 1986.

9 Meyer JE. New paradigm research in practice: the trials and tribulations of action research. *Journal of Advanced Nursing,* 1993;**18**:1066–72.

10 Webb C. Action research: philosophy, method and personal experiences. *Journal of Advanced Nursing* 1989;**14**:403–10.

11 Titchen A, Binnie A. Changing power relationships between nurses: a case study of early changes towards patient-centred nursing. *Journal of Clinical Nursing* 1993;**2**:219–29.

12 Elliott J. *Action research for educational change: developing teachers and teaching.* Milton Keynes: Open University Press, 1991.

13 Habermas J. *Knowledge and human interests.* London: Heinemann, 1972.

14 McNiff J. *Action research: principles and practice.* London: Macmillan Education Ltd, 1988.

15 Secretary of State for Health. *The new NHS: modern, dependable.* Cm 3807. London: The Stationery Office, 1997.

16 Rolfe G. *Expanding nursing knowledge: understanding and researching your own practice.* Oxford: Butterworth Heineman, 1998.

17 Carey LM, Matyas TA, Oke LE. Sensory loss in stroke patients: effective training of tactile and proprioceptive discrimination. *Archives of Physical Medicine and Rehabilitation* 1993;**74**:602–11.

18 Stark S. A nurse tutor's experience of personal and professional growth through action research. *Journal of Advanced Nursing* 1994;**19**(3):579–84.

19 Titchen A, Binnie A. What am I meant to be doing? Putting practice into theory and back again in new nursing roles. *Journal of Advanced Nursing* 1993;**18**:1054–65.

20 Meyer J, Bridges J. *An action research study into the organisation of care of older people in the accident and emergency department.* London: City University, 1998.

21 Lyon J. Applying Hart and Bond's typology; implementing clinical supervision in an acute setting. *Nurse Researcher* 1999;**6**:39–53.

22 Meyer JE. Action research in health-care practice: nature, present concerns and future possibilities. *NT Research* 1997;**2**:175–84.

23 Somekh B. Inhabiting each other's castles: towards knowledge and mutual growth though collaboration. *Educational Action Research Journal* 1994;**2**(3):357–81.

24 Walshe K, Ham C, Appleby J. Given in evidence. *Health Service Journal* 1995;**105**:28–9.

25 East L, Robinson J. Change in process: bringing about change in health care through action research. *Journal of Clinical Nursing* 1994;**3**:57–61.

26 Berger A. Why doesn't audit work? *Br Med J* 1998;**316**:875–6.

27 Ong BN. *The practice of health services research.* London: Chapman & Hall, 1993:65–82.

28 Ong BN. *Rapid appraisal and health policy.* London: Chapman & Hall, 1996.

29 Meyer JE. Lay participation in care: a challenge for multi-disciplinary teamwork. *Journal of Interprofessional Care* 1993;**7**:57–66.

30 Meyer JE. Lay participation in care: threat to the status quo. In: Wilson-Barnett J, Macleod Clark J. eds. *Research in health promotion and nursing.* London: Macmillan, 1993:86–100.

31 Brooking J. Patient and family participation in nursing care: the development of a nursing process measuring scale. London: University of London, unpublished PhD thesis, 1986.

32 Pankratz L, Pankratz D. Nursing autonomy and patients' rights: development of a nursing attitude scale. *Journal of Health and Social Behavior* 1974;**15**:211–16.

33 Citron MJ. Attitudes of nurses regarding the patients' role in the decision-making process and their implications for nursing education. *Dissertation Abstracts International* 1978;**38**:584.

34 Linn LS, Lewis CE. Attitudes towards self-care amongst practising physicians. *Medical Care* 1979;**17**:183–90.

35 Street A, Robinson A. Advanced clinical roles: investigating dilemmas and changing practice through action research. *Journal of Clinical Nursing* 1995;**4**:343–57.

8 Analysing qualitative data

CATHERINE POPE, SUE ZIEBLAND,
NICHOLAS MAYS

The nature of qualitative data

There is a widely held perception that qualitative research is small scale. As it tends to involve smaller numbers of subjects or settings than quantitative research it is assumed, incorrectly, that it generates fewer data than quantitative research. In fact, qualitative research can produce vast amounts of data.

As Chapters 2 to 4 have suggested, a range of different types of data may be collected during a qualitative study. These may include jotted notes, full field notes, interview and focus group transcripts and documentary material, as well as the researcher's own records of ongoing analytical ideas, research questions and the field diary, which provides a chronology of the events witnessed, and the progress of the research. These data are not necessarily small scale: transcribing a typical single qualitative interview generates a considerable amount of raw data – anything between 20 and 40 single-spaced pages of text.

Verbatim notes or audio/video tapes of face-to-face interviews or focus groups are transcribed to provide a record of what was said. The preparation of transcribed material will depend on the level of analysis being undertaken, but even if only sections of the data are intended for analysis, the preservation of the original recording tapes or documents is recommended. Transcribing is time consuming. Each hour of material can take six or seven hours to transcribe depending on the quality of the tape and the depth of information required. *Conversational analysis* of audio-taped material requires even more detailed annotation of a wide range of features of the talk studied, such as the exact length of pauses and the different types of emphasis in the spoken word. There are conventions for annotating transcripts for this purpose.[1] Even when the research is not concerned with analysing talk in this depth it is still important that the data provide an accurate record of what was said and done. The contribution of sighs, laughs and lengthy pauses should not be underestimated when analysing talk, and, as a minimum, these should be noted in the transcription.

Field notes of observational research contain detailed, highly descriptive accounts of several hours spent watching and listening, and often taking part in, events, interactions and conversations. This unprocessed experience needs to be transformed into notes, and from there into data that can be analysed. The jotted notes made in the field during an observational study need to be written up in full.

Whether using interviews or observation, the maintenance of meticulous records is vital – these are the raw data of the research. National qualitative data archives in Britain[2] have made secondary analysis of qualitative data possible, and mean that it is even more important that full records of qualitative studies are kept to allow the possibility of further analysis in the future.

The relationship between analysis and the data collected

Transcripts of interviews and field notes of observations provide a descriptive record, but they cannot provide explanations. The researcher has to make sense of the data by sifting and interpreting them. In much qualitative research the analytical process begins during the data collection phase as the data already gathered are analysed and fed into, or shape, the ongoing data collection. This is referred to as sequential analysis[3] or interim analysis[4] (see Figure 1). It allows the researcher to check and interpret the data she/he is collecting continually and to develop tentative conclusions based on the data already collected, or hypotheses for subsequent investigation in further data collection. Compared with quantitative methods, this has the advantage of allowing the researcher to go back and refine questions and to pursue emerging avenues of inquiry in further depth. Crucially, it also enables the researcher to look for deviant or negative cases; that is, examples of talk or events that run counter to the emerging propositions or hypotheses, in order to refine them. This type of continuous analysis is almost

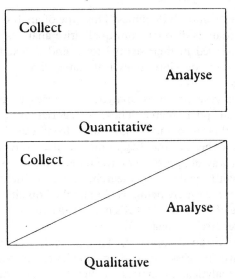

FIGURE 1—*Models of the research process*

inevitable in qualitative research; because the researcher is "in the field" collecting the data, it is impossible not to start thinking about what is being heard and seen.

The analysis

Although some of the initial analysis can be done whilst the data are being collected, as indicated above, there is still much to do once the researcher has left the field. Textual data, whether in the form of observational field notes or interview transcripts, are explored using some variant of *content analysis*. The most straight-forward type of content analysis is quantitative. This uses an unambiguous, predefined coding system and produces counts or frequencies that may be tabulated and analysed using standard statistical techniques. This approach is often used in media and mass communications studies. In general, qualitative research does not seek to quantify data, although simple counts can be useful in qualitative studies. One useful example of this approach is Silverman's research on communication in clinics.[5] This quantified features such as consultation length and the patient's use of questions and combined this information with the qualitative analysis to confirm a series of propositions about the differences between private and NHS clinics. This type of analysis that counts items in the data is distinct from qualitative analyses in which the data are preserved in their textual form and indexed in order to generate and/or develop analytical categories and theoretical explanations.

Qualitative research uses analytic categories to describe and explain social phenomena. These categories may be derived inductively, that is obtained gradually from the data, or used deductively, either at the beginning or part way through the analysis as a way of approaching the data. Though less commonly associated with qualitative research, more deductive forms of analysis are increasingly being used in applied qualitative research; one example of this is the SCPR's *framework approach*[6] (see Applied qualitative research on page 85).

Glaser and Strauss[7] coined the term *grounded theory* to describe the inductive process of coding incidents in the data and identifying analytical categories as they "emerge from" the data (developing hypotheses from the "ground" or research field upwards rather defining them *a priori*). This process involves identifying a theme and attempting to verify, confirm and qualify it by searching through the data. Once all data that match that theme have been located, the researcher repeats the process to identify further themes or categories.

The first stage in this process involves annotating or marking up themes in the field notes or interview transcripts. This is sometimes referred to as "coding", although it does not involve assigning numerical codes in the quantitative sense (where exclusive variables are defined and given preset codes or values). To avoid confusion the term "indexing" may be preferred.

Indexing qualitative data is a lengthy and sometimes tedious process. It requires reading and re-reading the material collected to identify themes and categories – these may centre on particular phrases, incidents or types of behaviour. Sometimes interesting or unfamiliar terms used by the group studied can form the basis of analytical categories. Becker and Geer's classic study of medical school training uncovered the specialised use of the term "crock" to denote patients who were seen as less worthwhile to treat by medical staff and students.[8]

All the data relevant to each category are identified and examined using a process called constant comparison, in which each item is checked or compared with the rest of the data to

establish analytical categories. Again, this requires a coherent and systematic approach. The process of indexing focus group or interview material may include searching for particular types of narrative – such as jokes or anecdotes, or types of interaction such as questions, challenges, censorship or changes of mind. The key point to note about this indexing process is that it is inclusive; categories are added to reflect as many of the nuances in the data as possible, rather than reducing them to a few numerical codes. It is also to be expected that sections of the data – such as discrete incidents – will include multiple themes and are thus coded using several categories. It is, therefore, important to have some system of cross-indexing that allows the analysis of data items which fit into more than one category. A number of computer software packages have been developed to facilitate this aspect of the analytical process (see Software packages designed to handle qualitative data on page 80).

The process of indexing the data creates a large number of what Perry calls "fuzzy categories"[9] or units. At this stage, there is likely to be considerable overlap and repetition between the categories. Informed by the analytical and theoretical ideas developed during the research, these categories are further refined and reduced in number by grouping them together. It is then possible to select key themes or categories for further investigation. In the study mentioned earlier, Becker and Geer pursued the use of the term "crock" by medical students to see what types of patients it described and when and how it was used. This meant collating all the instances when "crock" occurred in the data. Using these data, Becker and Geer were able to explain how medical students and staff categorised patients according to their utility for teaching/learning purposes. Once this was established, it became clear why "crocks" (typically the elderly patient, or the homeless alcoholic) who offered little or no possibility for learning about new or challenging disorders, were treated with disdain.

Grouping categories together typically entails a process of cutting and pasting, that is selecting sections of data on like or related themes and putting them together. The mechanics of how to do this vary. In the past, multiple copies of notes or transcripts were used so that sections could be, literally, cut out and pasted next to each other or sorted into different piles. Cardex systems have also been used – writing out relevant chunks of data onto index cards that could then be grouped in a card filing system.[10] It is also possible to create matrices or spreadsheets to facilitate this process of identifying themes. Whilst considered somewhat old-fashioned, this repeated physical contact and handling of the data has much to recommend it; the process of re-reading the data and sorting it into categories means that the researcher develops an intimate knowledge of the data, even if the process is laborious.

Word processors can be enormously helpful in searching large amounts of text for specific terms. While it is unlikely to be the sole focus of a qualitative research project, the simple frequency with which particular words or phrases appear in a piece of text can be illuminating. Word processing functions can offer considerable advantages to researchers who traditionally would have used annotations in the margins of field notes or interview transcripts, coloured pens, scissors and glue, card systems and paper files. By typing index terms directly into the computer file containing the textual data the "search" function can be used to gather chunks of text, which can then be copied and pasted. The split screen functions make this a particularly appealing method for sorting and copying data into separate analytic files.

Software packages designed to handle qualitative data

There are now several software packages that have been specifically designed for qualitative data analysis. Among the most widely used are QSR NUD*IST[11] and ATLAS/Ti.[12] The evolution of analytical software has been welcomed as an important development with the potential to improve the rigour of analysis.[13]

The current software offers functions that enable more complex organisation and retrieval of data than is possible within word processing packages. Software packages that have been designed to assist in the analysis of unstructured textual data all have code and retrieval functions and several other uses that will be recognisable to researchers. These include the ability to conduct selective retrievals and examine reports separately by any other indexing term (for example, the respondent's use of a particular term or a shared characteristic such as gender); to use algorithms to identify co-occurring codes in a range of logically overlapping or nesting possibilities; to attach annotations to sections of the text as "memos"; to add new codes; and to join together existing codes.

Most of the packages also provide counts of code frequencies and indicators of how many of the documents (for example interview transcripts) contain specific codes or indexing terms. While such counts may, on occasion, be illuminating to the researcher, it is important to treat them with caution. The reasons for this may be illustrated by contrasting the objectives of qualitative research with that of surveys and trials. In a study where everyone within a given population has had an equal chance of being selected to participate (this assumption is the cornerstone of sampling theory) and all respondents have been asked the same questions in the same manner, it is usually helpful to report responses as frequencies and percentages (relative frequencies). Surveys are designed to recruit sufficient numbers to represent the whole population. Trials aim to randomise enough subjects so that significant differences between treatment and control groups can be identified. By contrast, the qualitative methods of interviewing and observation are intended to identify subjective meanings and generate theory, which means that data collection will often continue until a saturation point has been reached (and no new categories are being contributed by the data), rather than until the sample is large enough to be considered statistically representative. In a qualitative study where the sample has not been (and often cannot be) selected to be numerically representative of the population, and where the interview technique is flexible and responsive, it can be misleading to report relative frequencies. This particularly applies if the questions have not been asked of all respondents, or have not been phrased in the same way or delivered at the same stage in the interview.

The ability to index, gather and sort are all important functions for organising and accessing the data, but these are only the initial stages in qualitative analysis. It has been suggested that computer-assisted analysis can help the researcher to build theoretical links, search for exceptions and examine "crucial cases" where counter evidence might be anticipated. A systematic search for "disconfirming evidence" can be assisted by using Boolean operators (such as or, and, not) to examine the data. An examination of the context of the fragments may be achieved either through considering which other index terms are attached to the data or by displaying the immediate context of the extract by including the lines of text that surround it. This function should particularly appeal to researchers who are concerned about the "decontextualisation" that can result from fragmenting the data into coded chunks. The Hypersoft package[14] uses what the developer calls "hyperlinks" to capture the conceptual links that are observed between sections of the data, thereby protecting the narrative structure from being fragmented.

There are many potential benefits of using a software package to help with the more laborious side of textual analysis, but some caution is advisable. Those who are used to the sampling methods used in surveys and trials are sometimes concerned that qualitative samples are small and unrepresentative. The prospect of computer-assisted analysis may persuade researchers (or those who fund them) that they can manage much larger amounts of data and increase the apparent "power" of their study. Qualitative studies, which are not designed to be representative in terms of how far they may be generalised statistically, may gain little from an expanded sample size except a more cumbersome dataset. The nature and size of the sample should be directed by the research question and analytic requirements, not by the available software. In some circumstances, a single case study design may be the most successful way of generating theory. Lee and Fielding[15] warn against the assumption that using a computer package will make analysis less time consuming, although it is hoped that it may make the process more demonstrably systematic.

Taking the analysis forward – the role of the researcher

The essential tasks of studying the text, recognising and refining the concepts and coding the data are inescapably the work of the researcher. For these reasons, it is important to dispel the notion that software packages are designed to deliver qualitative analysis of textual data. A computer package may be a useful aid when gathering together chunks of data, establishing links between the fragments, organising and reorganising the display and helping to find exceptions, but no package is capable of perceiving a link or defining an appropriate structure for the analysis. To take the analysis beyond the most basic descriptive and counting exercise requires the researcher's analytical skills in moving towards hypotheses or propositions about the data.

One way of performing this next stage is called *analytic induction*. Linked to grounded theory this involves an iterative testing and re-testing of theoretical ideas using the data. Bloor[16] describes in some detail how he used this procedure to reconstruct the decision-making rules used by ear, nose and throat surgeons (see Box 1). In essence, the researcher examines a set of cases, develops hypotheses or constructs and examines further cases to test these propositions – not unlike the statistical tests of association used in quantitative research.

In qualitative research, indexing the data and developing analytical categories tend to be carried out by a single researcher. However, some qualitative researchers have given attention to the notion that qualitative analyses may carry greater weight when they can be shown to be consistent between researchers (particularly when they have been undertaken to inform policy makers). This is close to the concept of inter-rater reliability, which is familiar in quantitative research. For example, Perry's study of patients with multiple sclerosis,[9] Daly et al.'s study of cardiac diagnosis,[17] and Waitzkin[18] used more than one analyst in order to improve their analyses. However, the appropriateness of the concept of inter-rater reliability in qualitative research is contested. Some qualitative researchers claim that a qualitative account cannot be

---

Box 1—Analysis

Stages in the analysis of field notes in a qualitative study of ear, nose and throat surgeons' disposal decisions for children referred for possible tonsillectomy and adenoidectomy (T&A)[16]

(1) Provisional classification—For each surgeon all cases categorised according to the disposal category used (for example, T&A or tonsillectomy alone)

(2) Identification of provisional case features—Common features of cases in each disposal category identified (for example, most T&A cases found to have three main clinical signs present)

(3) Scrutiny of deviant cases—Include in (2) or modify (1) to accommodate deviant cases (for example, T&A performed when only two of three signs present)

(4) Identification of shared case features—Features common to other disposal categories (history of several episodes of tonsillitis, for example)

(5) Derivation of surgeons' decision rules—From the common case features (for example, case history more important than physical examination)

(6) Derivation of surgeons' search procedures (for each decision rule)—The particular clinical signs looked for by each surgeon

Repeat (2) to (6) for each disposal category

held straightforwardly to represent the social world (just as all research findings reflect the identity of the researcher and the multiple nature of so called "reality"), thus different researchers are bound to offer different accounts. Another, less radical, assertion is that each researcher has unique insights into the data, which cannot be straightforwardly checked by others.[19]

In a recent contribution to the methodological debate, Armstrong et al.[20] attempted to answer a simpler empirical question: do qualitative researchers show consistency in their accounts of the same raw data? To test this, they asked six experienced qualitative researchers independently to analyse a single focus group transcript and to identify and rank the major themes emerging in the discussion. Another social scientist, who had not read the transcript of the focus group, then read the six reports in order to determine the main themes and to judge the extent to which the six researchers agreed. There was quite close agreement about the identity of the basic themes, but the six researchers "packaged" or linked and contextualised the themes differently. Armstrong et al. concluded that such reliability testing was limited by the inherent nature of the process of qualitative data analysis. On the other hand, the interpretations of the six researchers had much in common despite the fact that they were from both Britain and the United States and from more than one discipline (anthropology, psychology and sociology). By deliberately selecting a diverse range of analysts (albeit all experienced), Armstrong et al. constructed a tough test of inter-rater agreement and one which would be unusual in a typical research study. It would be interesting to see the same exercise repeated with quantitative data and analysis and analysts from three different social science disciplines!

Despite the potential limitations of the term "reliability" in the context of qualitative research highlighted by Armstrong et al., there may be merit in involving more than one analyst in situations where researcher bias is especially likely to be perceived to be a problem; for example, where social scientists are investigating the work of clinicians. In a study of the contribution of the use of echocardiography to the social process of diagnosing patients with suspected cardiac abnormalities, Daly et al. developed a modified form of qualitative analysis involving the sociologist researchers and the cardiologists who had managed the patients. The raw data consisted of transcripts of the consultations between the patients and the cardiologists, cardiologists' responses to a structured questionnaire and transcripts of open-ended research interviews with the cardiologists and with the patients.

First, the transcripts and questionnaire data were analysed by the researchers in order to make sense of the process of diagnosis, including the purpose of the test. From this analysis, the researchers identified the main aspects of the consultations that appeared to be related to the use of echocardiography. Next, these aspects or features of the clinical process were turned into criteria in relation to which other analysts could generate their own assessments of the meaning of the raw data. The cardiologists involved then independently assessed each case using the raw data in order to produce an account of how and why a test was or was not ordered and with what consequences. The assessments of the cardiologists and sociologists were compared statistically and the level of agreement was shown to be good. Finally, in cases where there was disagreement between the original researchers' analysis and that of the cardiologist, a further researcher repeated the analysis. Remaining discrepancies were resolved by consensus after discussion between the researchers and the cardiologists.

Although there was an element of circularity in part of this lengthy process (in that the formal criteria used by the cardiologists were derived from the initial researchers' analysis) and it involved the derivation of quantitative gradings and statistical analysis of inter-rater agreement, which are unusual in a qualitative study, it meant that clinical critics could not argue that the findings were simply based on the subjective judgements of an individual researcher.

Applied qualitative research

Similar considerations arise in other areas where qualitative methods are deployed. One approach to qualitative analysis known as the *framework approach* has been developed in Britain specifically for applied or policy relevant qualitative research in which the objectives of the investigation are typically set in advance and shaped by the information requirements of the funding body (for example, a health authority) rather than emerging from a reflexive research process. The timescales of applied research also tend to be shorter than more "basic" social research and there tends to be a need to link the qualitative analysis to findings from quantitative investigation. For these reasons, although the framework approach is heavily based in the original accounts and observations of the people studied (that is, "grounded" and inductive), it starts deductively from the aims and objectives already set for the study. It is systematic and designed so that the analytic process and interpretations can be viewed and assessed by people other than the primary analyst.

Box 2—The five stages of data analysis using the framework approach

- *Familiarisation* – immersion in the raw data (or typically a pragmatic selection from the data) by listening to tapes, reading transcripts, studying notes and so on, in order to list key ideas and recurrent themes
- *Identifying a thematic framework* – identifying all the key issues, concepts and themes by which the data can be examined and referenced. This is carried out by drawing on *a priori* issues and questions derived from the aims and objectives of the study as well as issues raised by the respondents themselves and views or experiences that recur in the data. The end product of this stage is a detailed index of the data, which labels the data into manageable chunks for subsequent retrieval and exploration
- *Indexing* – applying the thematic framework or index systematically to all the data in textual form by annotating the transcripts with numerical codes from the index, usually supported by short text descriptors to elaborate the index heading. Single passages of text can often encompass a large number of different themes each of which has to be recorded, usually in the margin of the transcript
- *Charting* – rearranging the data according to the appropriate part of the thematic framework to which they relate and forming charts. For example, there is likely to be a chart for each key subject area or theme with entries for several respondents. Unlike simple cut and paste methods that group verbatim text, the charts contain distilled summaries of views and experiences. Thus the charting process involves a considerable amount of abstraction and synthesis
- *Mapping and interpretation* – using the charts to define concepts, map the range and nature of phenomena, create typologies and find associations between themes with a view to providing explanations for the findings. The process of mapping and interpretation is influenced by the original research objectives as well as by the themes that have emerged from the data themselves.

The topic guide used to collect data under the framework approach (for example, to guide depth interviews) tends to be more structured from the outset than would be the norm for much other qualitative research. The transcription process is followed by five stages of analysis, which are similar to the steps in more conventional qualitative analysis discussed in this chapter. However, they tend to be more explicit and more strongly informed by a priori reasoning[6] (see Box 2). Framework analysis is most commonly used with individual interview or focus group data. It is easy to see, even with a summary of the five stages, how laborious thorough qualitative data analysis can be.

Conclusion

This chapter has shown that analysing qualitative data is not a simple or quick task. Done properly, it is systematic and rigorous, and therefore labour intensive for the researcher(s) involved and time consuming. Fielding contends that "good qualitative analysis is able to document its claim to reflect some of the truth of a phenomenon by reference to systematically gathered data", in contrast, "poor qualitative analysis is anecdotal, unreflective, descriptive without being focused on a coherent line of inquiry".[21] At its heart, good qualitative analysis relies on the skill, vision and integrity of the researcher doing that analysis, and as Dingwall et al. have pointed out, this may require highly trained and, crucially, experienced researchers.[22]

Further reading

Bryman A, Burgess R. eds. Analysing qualitative data. London: Routledge, 1993.
Miles M, Huberman A. Qualitative data analysis. London: Sage, 1984.

References

1 Heritage J. Garfinkel and ethnomethodology. Cambridge: Polity, 1984.
2 E.S.R.C. QUALIDATA: Qualitative Data Archival Resource Centre, established 1994, University of Essex.
3 Becker HS. Sociological work. London: Allen Lane, 1971.
4 Miles M, Huberman A. Qualitative data analysis. London: Sage, 1984.
5 Silverman D. Going private: ceremonial forms in a private oncology clinic. Sociology 1984;18:191–202.
6 Ritchie J, Spencer L. Qualitative data analysis for applied policy research. In Bryman A, Burgess R. eds. Analysing qualitative data. London: Routledge, 1993:173–94.

7 Glaser BG, Strauss AL. *The discovery of grounded theory.* Chicago, IL: Aldine, 1967.
8 Becker HS, Geer B. Participant observation: the analysis of qualitative field data. In: Burgess RG. *Field research: a sourcebook and field manual.* London: Allen and Unwin, 1982.
9 Perry S. *Living with multiple sclerosis.* Aldershot: Avebury, 1994.
10 Scambler G, Hopkins A. Accommodating epilepsy in families. In: Anderson R, Bury M. eds. *Living with chronic illness: the experience of patients.* London: Unwin Hyman, 1988.
11 Richards T, Richards L. QSR NUD*IST V3.0. London: Sage, 1994.
12 Muhr T. ATLAS/Ti for Windows, 1996.
13 Kelle U. ed. *Computer-aided qualitative data analysis: theory, methods and practice.* London: Sage, 1995.
14 Dey I. *Qualitative data analysis: A user friendly guide for Social Scientists.* London: Routledge, 1993.
15 Lee R, Fielding N. User's experiences of qualitative data analysis software. In: Kelle U. ed. *Computer aided qualitative data analysis: theory, methods and practice.* London: Sage, 1995.
16 Bloor M. On the analysis of observational data: a discussion of the worth and uses of inductive techniques and respondent validation. *Sociology* 1978;**12**:545–52.
17 Daly J, McDonald I, Willis E. Why don't you ask them? A qualitative research framework for investigating the diagnosis of cardiac normality. In: Daly J, McDonald I, Willis E, eds. *Researching health care: designs, dilemmas, disciplines.* London: Routledge, 1992:189–206.
18 Waitzkin H. *The politics of medical encounters.* New Haven: Yale University Press, 1991.
19 Morse JM. Designing funded qualitative research. In: Denzin NK, Lincoln YS, eds. *Handbook of qualitative research.* London: Sage, 1994:220–35.
20 Armstrong D, Gosling A, Weinman J, Marteau T. The place of inter-rater reliability in qualitative research: an empirical study. *Sociology* 1997;**31**:597–606.
21 Fielding N. Ethnography. In Fielding N. ed. *Researching social life.* London: Sage, 1993: 155–71(168–9).
22 Dingwall R, Murphy E, Watson P, Greatbatch D, Parker S. Catching goldfish: quality in qualitative research. *Journal of Health Services Research and Policy* 1998;**3**:167–72.

9 Quality in qualitative health research

NICHOLAS MAYS, CATHERINE POPE

Introduction

This book has outlined the main methods used in qualitative research and described some of the ways in which these methods have been applied to answer questions about health and health care. As noted in Chapter 1, qualitative methods have long been used in the social sciences, but their use in health and health care settings is comparatively recent. In the last decade, qualitative methods have appeared in areas such as health services research and health technology assessment, and there has been a corresponding rise in the reporting of qualitative research studies in medical and related journals.[1] Interest in these methods and their wider exposure in the field of health research has led to necessary scrutiny of qualitative research. Researchers from other traditions are increasingly concerned to understand qualitative methods and, most importantly, to examine the claims researchers make about the findings obtained from these methods.

Qualitative research in health and health services has had to overcome prejudice and a number of misunderstandings. For example, some people believe that qualitative research is "easy" – a soft option that requires no skills or training. In fact, the opposite is more likely to be the case. The data generated by qualitative studies are cumbersome and difficult to analyse[2] and their analysis requires a high degree of interpretative skill. Qualitative research also suffers from the "stigma of the small n"[3] because it tends to deal with a small number of settings or respondents and does not seek to be statistically representative. However, in expert hands this feature is irrelevant to the strength of the approach.

Nonetheless, the status of all forms of research depends on assessing the quality of the methods used. In the field of qualitative research, concern about assessing quality has manifested itself recently in the proliferation of guidelines for doing and judging qualitative work.[2,4-6] Those using and funding research have played an important role in the development of these guidelines as they become increasingly familiar with qualitative methods, but require some means of assessing their quality and of distinguishing "good" and "poor" quality research. To this end, the NHS Research and Development Programme recently funded a review of qualitative research methods relevant to health technology assessment.[7] However, while the sponsors of this review may have hoped for a small set of simple quality guidelines to emerge, any thoughtful analysis of the issue is inevitably far more complex.

The issue of "quality" in qualitative research is part of a much larger and contested debate about the nature of the knowledge produced by qualitative research, whether its quality can legitimately be judged and, if so, how. The chapters of this book have touched on a number of issues related to the quality of qualitative research. In outlining some of the most frequently used qualitative methods and demonstrating their contemporary application in health research, each chapter has referred to the strengths and limitations of particular methods. In doing this, each author clearly had some notion of quality in mind.

This chapter attempts to bring together some of these quality issues, although it cannot do full justice to the wider epistemological debate. It outlines two views of how qualitative methods might be judged. It goes on to argue that qualitative research can be assessed with reference to the same broad criteria as quantitative research, albeit differently used, and that two main criteria of quality in qualitative research stand out – validity and relevance.[8] The chapter concludes with a list of questions that might be used to begin to assess the quality of a piece of qualitative research. The list is designed simply to indicate some of the questions worth considering when evaluating qualitative research, and not as a definitive inventory.

Can we use the same quality criteria for qualitative and quantitative research? Two opposing answers

There has been considerable debate among qualitative researchers over whether qualitative and quantitative methods can and should be assessed according to the same quality criteria. The debate is complex because there is an underlying lack of consensus about precisely what qualitative research is and the variety of approaches included under this heading. Other than the total rejection of any quality criteria, it is possible to identify two broad, opposing positions.[8] First, there are those who have argued that qualitative research in all its guises represents a distinctive paradigm that generates a different type of knowledge from quantitative research. Therefore, different quality criteria should apply. Second, there are those who have argued that there is no separate philosophy of knowledge underpinning qualitative research and so the same criteria should be applied to qualitative and quantitative research. Within each position, it is possible to see a range of views.

Separate and different: the anti-realist position

Advocates of this position argue that since qualitative research represents a distinct paradigm that generates a distinct form of knowledge, it is inappropriate to apply criteria derived from an alternative paradigm. This means that qualitative research cannot and should not be judged by conventional measures of validity (the test of whether the research is true to some underlying reality), generalisability (the degree to which the specifics of the research can be applied more widely to other settings and populations) and reliability (the extent to which the same findings are produced by repeating the research procedures). For those who adopt this anti-realist position, it would also be inappropriate to use mixed or multiple methods in the same study.

At the core of this position is a rejection of what Lincoln and Guba[9] call "naïve realism" – a belief that there is a single, unequivocal social reality or truth that is entirely independent of the researcher and of the research process. Instead, they suggest "'truth' is defined as the best informed . . . and most sophisticated . . . construction on which there is consensus (although there may be several constructions extant which simultaneously meet that criterion) . . . the inquirer and the inquired are interlocked in such a way that the findings of an investigation are the *literal creation* of the inquiry process."[9]

There are still more extreme relativists who hold that there is no basis even for the consensus referred to by Guba and Lincoln and that all research perspectives are unique and each is equally valid in its own terms. The absence of any external standards would clearly make it impossible for one researcher to judge another's research. Yet, as Murphy *et al.* note, in health services research such a relativist position precludes qualitative research from deriving any unequivocal insights relevant to action and would, therefore, command little support among applied health researchers.[7]

Those relativists who maintain that separate criteria are required to evaluate qualitative research have put forward a range of different assessment schemes. In part, this is because the choice and relative importance of different criteria of quality depend on the topic and the purpose of the research. If the key question for qualitative researchers is: "Why do people do what they do?" then for Popay *et al.* research quality relates to the sampling strategy, adequacy of theory, collection and analysis of data, the extent to which the context has been understood, and whether the knowledge generated incorporates an understanding of the nature of subjective meanings in their social contexts.[10] While there may be some broad similarities between quality standards in quantitative and qualitative research, the fundamental differences in the knowledge each approach generates require that quality is assessed differently in the two traditions.[11]

Hammersley has attempted to pull together the different quality criteria and concerns of the relativists (or anti-realists), as follows:[8]

- The degree to which substantive and formal theory is produced and the degree of development of such theory
- The novelty of the claims made from the theory
- The consistency of the theoretical claims with the empirical data collected
- The credibility of the account to those studied and to readers
- The extent to which the description of the culture of the setting provides a basis for competent performance in the culture studied
- The extent to which the findings are transferable to other settings
- The reflexivity of the account – that is, the degree to which the effects of the research strategies on the findings are assessed and/or the amount of information about the research process that is provided to readers.

These criteria are open to challenge. For example, it is arguable whether all research should be concerned to develop theory. At the same time, many of the criteria listed are not exclusive to qualitative research (for example, the extent to which findings are transferable), suggesting that there is a case for assessing both qualitative and quantitative research against the same standards, even if that assessment has to be tailored to the type of research used.

Using criteria from quantitative research: subtle realism

Authors such as Hammersley[12] and Kirk and Miller[13] agree that all research involves subjective perceptions and observations, and that different methods will produce different pictures of the social phenomena being studied. However, unlike the anti-realists, they argue that this does not mean that we cannot believe in the existence of phenomena independent of our claims about them; that is, there is some underlying reality that may be studied. The role of qualitative and quantitative research is to attempt to represent that reality rather than to imagine that "the truth" can be attained. Hammersley refers to this as *subtle realism*.

The logic of this position is that there are ways to assess the different perspectives offered by different research processes against each other and against criteria of quality common to both qualitative and quantitative research, particularly those of validity and relevance.[8] However, the means of assessment may be modified to take account of the distinctive goals of qualitative research. For example, qualitative research frequently does not seek to generalise to a wider population for predictive purposes, but seeks to understand specific behaviour in a naturally occurring context. Similarly, reliability, as conventionally defined, may be of little relevance if unique situations cannot be reconstructed or if the setting studied is undergoing considerable social change.[14]

A comprehensive review of the literature on qualitative research in health technology assessment[7] concluded by supporting Hammersley's case[8] for assessing such research according to its validity, defined as the extent to which the account accurately represented the social phenomena to which it referred, and its relevance, defined in terms of the capacity of the research to help some group of practitioners solve the problems they faced. Each broad criterion will be discussed in turn.

Assessing the validity of qualitative research

There are no mechanical or "easy" solutions to limit the likelihood that there will be errors in qualitative research. However, there are various ways of improving validity, each of which requires the exercise of judgement on the part of researcher and reader.

Triangulation

Triangulation involves the comparison of the results from either two or more different methods of data collection (for example interviews and observation) or, more simply, from two or more data sources (for example, interviews with members of different interest groups). The researcher looks for patterns of convergence to develop or corroborate an overall interpretation. Triangulation is generally accepted as a means of ensuring the comprehensiveness of a set of findings. It is more controversial as a genuine test of the truthfulness or validity of a study. The latter test relies on the assumption that any weaknesses in one method will be compensated by strengths in another. Occasionally, qualitative methods will reveal inadequacies in quantitative measures or show that quantitative results are at odds with observed behaviour. For example, Stone and Campbell's depth interviews in Nepal (mentioned in Chapter 1) revealed very different attitudes towards abortion and family planning from those recorded in formal fertility surveys.[15] Similarly, Meyer's multi-method approach highlighted the gap between the findings derived from attitudinal scales and everyday talk about, and practice in relation to, lay participation in care on the ward she studied[16] (see Chapter 7). However, this use of triangulation is contested. Silverman argues that data from different sources can only be used to identify the context-specific nature of differing accounts and behaviour.[17] He points out that discrepancies between different data sources (such as from doctors and their patients) present a problem of adjudication between rival accounts. Thus, triangulation may be better seen as a way of making a study more comprehensive, or of encouraging a more *reflexive* analysis of the data (see Reflexivity on page 96) than as a pure test of validity.

Respondent validation

Respondent validation, or member checking as it is sometimes called, includes a range of techniques in which the investigator's account is compared with the accounts of those who have been investigated in order to establish the level of correspondence between the two sets. The reactions of those studied to the analyses are then incorporated into the study findings. Lincoln and Guba[9] regard respondent validation as the strongest available check on the credibility of a research project. However, there are limitations to these techniques as validation tests. For example, the account produced by the researcher is designed for a wide audience and will, inevitably, be different from the account of an individual informant simply because of their different roles in the research process. As a result, it is better to think of respondent validation as part of a process of error reduction, which also generates further original data, which, in turn, require interpretation.[18]

Clear exposition of methods of data collection and analysis

Since the methods used in research unavoidably influence the objects of enquiry (and qualitative researchers are particularly aware of this), it is important to provide a clear account of the process of data collection and analysis. This is so that readers can judge the evidence upon which conclusions are drawn, taking account of the way that the evidence was gathered. For example, in an observational study, it would be particularly pertinent to document the period of time over which observations were made and the depth or quality of the researcher's access to the research setting.

A common failing of qualitative research reports is an inadequate account of the process of data analysis. This is compounded by the inductive nature of much qualitative work in which prior conceptualisation is largely inappropriate since concepts and categories are developed through the process of undertaking the research. As a result, the processes of data collection and analysis are frequently interwoven. Nonetheless, by the end of the study, it should be possible to provide a clear account of how early, simpler systems of classification evolved into more sophisticated coding structures and thence into clearly defined concepts and explanations for the data collected. In some situations, it may be appropriate to assess the inter-rater reliability of coding by asking another researcher independently to code some of the raw data using coding criteria previously agreed. Where this is not feasible or appropriate (see Chapter 8 for more on this), it may be preferable to show that a range of potential explanations has been explored to make sense of the data collected. Finally, it is important to include in the written account sufficient data to allow the reader to judge whether the interpretation offered is adequately supported by the data. This is one of the reasons why qualitative research reports are generally longer than those of quantitative studies since it can be difficult to summarise the data that support a concept or explanation.

Reflexivity

Reflexivity means sensitivity to the ways in which the researcher and the research process have shaped the data collected, including the role of prior assumptions and experience, which can influence even the most avowedly inductive enquiries. Researchers can keep a personal research diary alongside the data collection and analysis in which to record their reactions to events occurring during the period of the research. They can and should make their personal and intellectual biases plain at the outset of any research reports to enhance the credibility of their findings. The effects of personal characteristics such as age, gender, social class and professional status (for example that of doctor, nurse, physiotherapist, sociologist, etc.) on the data collected and the "distance" between the researcher and those researched also need to be discussed.

Attention to negative cases

As well as exploring alternative explanations for the data collected, a long-established tactic for reducing error is to search for, and discuss, elements in the data that contradict, or appear to contradict, the emerging explanation of the phenomena under study. *Deviant case analysis* helps refine the analysis until it can explain all or the vast majority of the cases under scrutiny. It is similar to Popper's quest for evidence that disproves established theories in the natural sciences and can help counteract some of the preconceptions that all researchers bring to their research. In this way, it can contribute to increasing the sophistication and credibility of research reports.[19] Another version of deviant or negative case analysis is to attempt to incorporate seemingly different findings from different studies into a more refined, overarching analysis.

Fair dealing

The final technique for reducing bias in qualitative research is to ensure that the research design explicitly incorporates a wide range of different perspectives so that the viewpoint of one group is never presented as if it represents the sole truth about any situation. Dingwall[20] coined the term "fair dealing" to describe this process of attempting to be non-partisan; for him, fair dealing marks the difference between social science and "muck-raking journalism". However, this concern to deal even-handedly with all those studied is not shared by all researchers. Indeed, there is a long tradition in sociology, dating from the 1930s Chicago School, of adopting the perspective of the "underdog" against the dominant views of powerful elites.[21] This position has been severely mauled in recent times: Strong scathingly described it as being more concerned with being "right on" than with being right.[22]

Relevance

Hammersley argued that good quality qualitative research had to be relevant in some way to a public concern, though this did not necessarily mean that the research should slavishly adhere to the immediate concerns or problems defined by policy makers, professionals or managers.[8] Research could be relevant when it either added to knowledge or increased the confidence with which existing knowledge was regarded. Another important dimension of relevance is the extent to which findings can be generalised beyond the setting in which they were generated. Quantitative researchers frequently criticise qualitative studies for their lack of representativeness. However, it is possible to use forms of probability sampling such as stratified sampling techniques in qualitative research in order to ensure that the range of settings chosen is representative of the population about which the researcher wishes to generalise. Another tactic is to ensure that the research report has sufficient descriptive detail for the reader to be able to judge whether or not the findings apply in other similar settings.

Finally, it has to be recognised that generalisation from qualitative research does not rely exclusively on notions of statistical logic. The extent to which inferences can be drawn from one setting to another depends as much on the adequacy of the explanatory theory on which they are based as on statistical representativeness.[19] Thus the test is whether categories of cases or settings that are theoretically similar behave in the same way rather than cases or settings that are substantively similar. One way of looking at this is to explore the extent to which the sample of cases studied included the full range of potentially relevant cases. This is *theoretical sampling* in which an initial sample is drawn to include as many as possible of the factors that might affect variability of behaviour, but is then extended, as required, in the light of early findings and emergent theory.[2] Under conceptual or theoretical sampling, statistical "minority" groups are frequently over-represented in order to test whether the emerging explanations are equally robust when applied to widely differing populations. The full sample, therefore, attempts to include the full range of settings relevant to the conceptualisation of the subject.

Is there any place for quality guidelines?

The hotly contested debate about whether quality criteria should be applied to qualitative research, together with the differences of view between "experts" about which criteria are appropriate and how they should be assessed, should warn against unthinking reliance on any one set of guidelines. A number of practical checklists have been published recently in the UK to help with judging the quality of qualitative work.[2,4,5] Indeed, a crude checklist was included in the previous edition of this book.[6] The checklists cover a wide range of issues that may potentially be relevant to the rigour of qualitative studies. However, following Hammersley[8] and the recent overview by Murphy *et al.*,[7] two central criteria of rigour stand out – validity and relevance. Neither criterion is straightforward to assess. Each requires judgements to be made. Thus, instead of setting out yet another set of guidelines, the final section of this chapter consists of some possible questions to ask of any piece of qualitative research with an emphasis on relevance and validity. The questions could also be used by researchers at different times during the life of a particular research project in order to improve its quality.

Some questions that might be asked of a qualitative study

• Worth/relevance
Was this piece of work worth doing at all? Has it contributed usefully to knowledge?

• Clarity of research question

If not at the outset of the study, by the end of the research process was the research question clear? Was the researcher able to set aside her/his research preconceptions?

• Appropriateness of the design to the question

Would a different method have been more appropriate? Did the study require the use of qualitative methods? For example, if a casual hypothesis was being tested, was a qualitative approach really appropriate?

• Context

Is the context/setting adequately described so that the reader can relate the findings to other settings?

• Sampling

Did the sample include the full range of possible cases/settings so that conceptual rather than statistical generalisations could be made (that is, more than convenience sampling)? If appropriate, were efforts made to obtain data that might contradict or modify the analysis by extending the sample (for example, to a different type of area)?

• Data collection and analysis

Were the data collection and analysis procedures systematic? Was an "audit trail" provided such that someone else could repeat each stage, including the analysis?

How well did the analysis succeed in incorporating all the observations? Was there unexplained variation? To what extent did the analysis develop concepts and categories capable of explaining key processes or respondents' accounts or observations? Was it possible to follow the iteration between data and the explanations for the data (theory)? Did the researcher seek disconfirming cases?

• Reflexivity of the account

Did the researcher self-consciously assess the likely impact of the methods used on the data obtained? Were sufficient data included in the report of the study to provide sufficient evidence for readers to assess whether analytical criteria had been met?

Conclusion

Although the issue of quality in qualitative health and health services research has received considerable attention, a recent paper was able to argue, legitimately, that "quality in qualitative research is a mystery to many health services researchers".[23] This chapter has tried to show how qualitative researchers endeavour to address the issue of quality in their research. It has outlined the broad debates about the nature of the knowledge produced by qualitative research and indicated some of the questions it is worth asking of a particular study or research report.

As in quantitative research, the basic strategy to ensure rigour, and thus quality, in qualitative research, is systematic, self-conscious research design, data collection, interpretation and communication. Qualitative research, as this book has shown, has much to offer. Its methods can, and do, enrich our knowledge of health and health care. It is not, however, an easy option or the route to a quick answer. As Dingwall et al. conclude, "qualitative research requires real skill, a combination of thought and practice and not a little patience."[23]

Further reading

Murphy E, Dingwall R, Greatbatch D, Parker S, Watson P. Qualitative research methods in health technology assessment: a review of the literature. *Health Technology Assessment* 1998:2(16).

Dingwall R, Murphy E, Watson P, Greatbatch D, Parker S. Catching goldfish: quality in qualitative research. *Journal of Health Services Research and Policy* 1998:3:167–72.

References

1 Harding G, Gantley M. Qualitative methods: beyond the cookbook. *Family Practice* 1998;**15**:76–9.
2 Boulton M, Fitzpatrick R. Qualitative methods for assessing health care. *Quality in Health Care* 1994;**3**:107–13.
3 Faltermaier T. Why public health research needs qualitative approaches: subjects and methods in change. *European Journal of Public Health* 1997;**7**:357–63.
4 Blaxter M. Criteria for evaluation of qualitative research. *Medical Sociology News* 1996;**22**:68–71.
5 Secker J, Wimbush E, Watson J, Milburn K. Qualitative methods in health promotion research: some criteria for quality. *Health Education Journal* 1995;**54**:74–87.
6 Mays N, Pope C. Rigour in qualitative research. In: Mays N, Pope C, eds. *Qualitative research in health care.* London: BMJ Books, 1996.
7 Murphy E, Dingwall R, Greatbatch D, Parker S, Watson P. Qualitative research methods in health technology assessment: a review of the literature. *Health Technology Assessment* 1998:2(16).

8 Hammersley M. *Reading ethnographic research.* New York: Longman, 1990.
9 Lincoln YS, Guba EG. *Naturalistic inquiry.* Newbury Park, CA: Sage, 1985:84.
10 Popay J, Rogers A, Williams G. Qualitative research and the gingerbread man. *Health Education Journal* 1995;**54**:389–443.
11 Popay J, Rogers A, Williams G. Rationale and standards for the systematic review of qualitative literature in HSR. *Qualitative Health Research* 1998;**8**:341–51.
12 Hammersley M. *What's wrong with ethnography?* London: Routledge, 1992.
13 Kirk J, Miller M. *Reliability and validity in qualitative research* Qualitative Research Methods Series No 1. London: Sage, 1986.
14 Seale C, Silverman D. Ensuring rigour in qualitative research. *European Journal of Public Health* 1997;**7**:379–84.
15 Stone L, Campbell JG. The use and misuse of surveys in international development: an experiment from Nepal. *Human Organisation* 1986;**43**:27–37.
16 Meyer JE. *Lay participation in care in a hospital setting: an action research study.* London: University of London, unpublished PhD thesis, 1995.
17 Silverman D. *Interpreting qualitative data: methods for analysing talk, text and interaction.* London: Sage, 1993.
18 Bloor M. Techniques of validation in qualitative research: a critical commentary. In: Miller G, Dingwall R, eds. *Context and method in qualitative research.* London: Sage, 1997:37–50.
19 Silverman D. Telling convincing stories: a plea for more cautious positivism in case studies. In: Glassner B, Moreno JD, eds. *The qualitative–quantitative distinction in the social sciences.* Dordrecht: Kluwer Academic, 1989:57–77.
20 Dingwall R. Don't mind him – he's from Barcelona: qualitative methods in health studies. In: Daly J, McDonald I, Willis E, eds. *Researching health care.* London: Tavistock/Routledge, 1992:161–75.
21 Guba EG, Lincoln YS. *Fourth generation evaluation.* Newbury Park, CA: Sage, 1989.
22 Strong P. Qualitative sociology in the UK. *Qualitative Sociology* 1988;**11**:13–28.
23 Dingwall R, Murphy E, Watson P, Greatbatch D, Parker S. Catching goldfish: quality in qualitative research. *Journal of Health Services Research and Policy* 1998;**3**:167–72.

Index

access, observational research 33–4
accident and emergency,
observational studies 32
accuracy, consensus methods 45
action research
contribution to social science
and social change 62–4
defined 59–60
democracy in 61–2
focus groups 22
in health care 68–72
participation in 60–1
types of 64–8
action-reflection spirals 61–2, 69
active interviews 16
admissions, observational study 33
agreement
action research 60
consensus methods 44–5
analysis *see* qualitative analysis
analytic induction 82–3
anonymity, consensus methods *41*
anti-realist position 91–3
applicability, consensus methods
45–6
applications, consensus methods
46–8
applied research 85–7
appropriateness
group work 24
research questions 99
attitudes, exploring 20, 27–8
audio taping
conversational analysis 75–6
group work 27
interviews 17

Boolean operators 81
business process re-engineering,
case study 54–5

Cardex systems 79–80
cardiology

observational studies 32
qualitative analysis 84–5
case study research 51–7
categories, qualitative research 37,
78–80
change, action research 63–4, 68–9
charting, framework approach *86*
Chicago School 31, 97
clarity, research questions 99
clinical interviews 12–13
clinicians, action research 68
coding 36, 78
communication, group work 21–2,
24
comparison, case study research
53
composition, focus groups 23–5
computer-assisted analysis 81–2
confidentiality, group work 22
congruence, observational research
37
consensus methods
applications 46–8
defined 40–1
described 41–3
methodological issues 43–5
validity and applicability 45–6
constant comparison 78–9
construct validity, case study
research 55–6
content analysis
observational research 37
textual data 77
context 99
control, in interviews 16
conventions, observational data 36
conversational analysis 75–6
covert research 35
critical incidents, recording data
36
criticism
in group work 23
of qualitative data 1
crocks 78, 79

crucial cases 81
cultural values, focus groups 22
cutting and pasting, data 79

data collection
    and analysis 76–80
    case study research 55–6
    exposition of 95–6
    focus groups 22
    questions about 99
    see also qualitative data
decision making, group 41
decontextualisation 81
deduction, in analysis 78
defamiliarising 4
Delphi process 41–2, 44, 46, 47,
    48
democracy, action research 61–2
depth interviews 12, 94
description, observational data 36
deviant case analysis 96
differences, in focus groups 26
directiveness, of interviewing
    techniques 15–16
disagreements, focus groups 26
disconfirming evidence 81
diversity, focus groups 24

ear, nose and throat (ENT),
    observational study 32
echocardiography 84–5
empirical evaluative studies 51
empowering action research 64,
    65–7, 68
ethics, observational research 35
ethnography 31
exercises, focus groups 26
experimental action research 64,
    65–7, 68

face-to-face interviews 8
fair dealing 97
familiarisation, framework
    approach 86
feedback
    action research 62
    consensus methods 41

field access, observational methods
    33–4
focus groups 8
    analysis and writing up 27
    conducting studies 23–5
    defined 20–3
    running sessions 25–7
framework approach 78, 85–7
fuzzy categories 79

gatekeepers 34
generalisations 63, 97
grounded theory 78, 82
group decision making 41
group interaction
    consensus development 48
    focus groups 20, 21
guidelines, quality 98

Handbook of Qualitative Research 2
Hawthorne effect 34–5
health care
    action research in 68–72
    focus groups 20–8
health care settings
    observational methods 30–8
    qualitative interviews 11–18
health research
    qualitative methods 1–9
    quality in qualitative 89–100
health services research
    case studies 50–7
    consensus methods 40–8
hierarchy, focus groups 24
homogeneity, focus groups 24
hospitals
    action research 69–71
    observational studies 33
hyperlinks 82
Hypersoft package 81–2

identification
    interviewees 18
    thematic framework 86
indexing 78–9, 86
inductive process 78
    see also analytic induction
inter-rater reliability 83–5

interim analysis 76–7
interpretation, framework
    approach *86*
interpretative research 3–4
interviewees
    identification of 18
    perceptions of researchers 15
interviews *see* qualitative interviews
introductory letters, to
    interviewees 18
iteration, consensus methods *41*

observational research 8, 30–1
    in health and health services
        31–3
    quality in 37–8
    recording 35–7
    theorising from 37
    using 33–5
opinions, exploring 27–8, 46
organisational action research 64,
    65–7
overtness, health care research 35

judgement, consensus
    development 48

Kappa statistic 44
knowledge, contribution of action
    research 63

lay participation, action research
    69–71

mapping, framework approach *86*
materials, for group discussion 26
measurement, in qualitative
    research 3
memory, observational research 35
misunderstandings
    qualitative interviews 13–14
    qualitative research 1–2, 89
multi-method approach 4, 94

naive realism 91
narrative, in indexing 79
naturalistic approach 4, 31
needs, exploring 20
negative case analysis 96
neurology, observational studies 32
NHS
    case study research 53–4
    observational studies 33
nominal group technique (NGT)
    41, 42–3, 46, 47, 48
notes
    action research 63
    observational research 35–6, 76
    recording interviews 17

participant observation 4
participants, consensus methods
    43–4
participation, action research 60–1
patient careers 31–2
perspectives
    adopting underdog 97
    change through group work
        22–3
pitfalls, in interviews 16–17
planning, consensus development
    47–8
policy research, case studies 50–7
politics, case study research 52
practitioner-led research 62–3
probability sampling 97
process gain 41
process loss 41
professionalising action research
    64, *65–7*
purchaser-provider contracting
    study 56
purposive sampling 33–4, 55

qualitative analysis
    exposition of 95–6
    focus groups 27
    observational data 36–7
    qualitative data 77–80
    questions about 99
    role of researcher 82–5
    see also computer-assisted
        analysis; framework approach;
        negative case analysis

qualitative data
   analysis and collection 76–80
   criticism of 1
   nature of 75–6
   software packages 80–2
   see also data collection; recording
qualitative interviews
   conducting 13–15
   recording 17
   researchers as research
     instruments 15–17
   types of 11–13
   see also interviewees
qualitative research
   applied 85–7
   assessing validity of 94–7
   criteria for assessment 90–3
   defined 3–5
   methods used 6–9
   questions about 98–9
   theory and method 1–3
   uses of 5–6
quality
   observational research 37–8
   qualitative health research
     89–100
quantitative analysis 77–8
quantitative research 3, 4–5, 6, 13,
   32, 90–3
questionnaires, group work 26–7
questions
   interviews 14
   on qualitative studies 98–9

Rapid Appraisal 69
recording
   action research 63
   observational data 35–7
   qualitative interviews 17
   see also qualitative data
records 76
reflexivity 96, 99
relevance 97–8
reliability 83–5
representativeness 36, 97
research instruments, researchers
   as 15–17
research methods 2
research questions 99

research strategy 2
researchers
   interviewees' perceptions 15
   observational methods 34–5
   as research instruments 15–17
   task of analysis 82–5
resource management case study
   53–4
respondent validation 94–5

sampling
   case study research 55
   focus groups 23–5
   observational methods 33–4
   qualitative interviews 18
   questions about 99
   see also probability sampling;
     theoretical sampling
self-reflective notes 63
semistructured interviews 12, 13
sequential analysis 76–7
skills 8, 35
software packages, qualitative data
   80–2
stand alone research 6
statistical group response,
   consensus methods *41*
statistics, consensus methods 45
structured eavesdropping 25
structured interviews 11–12
subtle realism 93
survey questionnaires 5–6, 23

taboo topics, group work 22
terminology 1–2
textual data, analysis 77
theoretical perspectives 2, 37
theoretical sampling 23, 98
theorising, observational research
   37
timetables, patient careers 31–2
total purchasing case study 53, 55
transcriptions
   audio material 17, 75
   framework approach 87
triangulation 55, 94
typology, action research 64–8

underdog perspective 97

validation, of quantitative research 6
validity
  anti-realist position 91
  case study research 55–6
  consensus methods 45–6

of qualitative research 94–7

Whyte's directiveness scale 15–16
word processors 80
wording
  qualitative interviews 14
  survey questionnaires 5–6, 23
worth, qualitative studies 98